Life and Breath

Life and Breath

[
Preventing, Treating, and Reversing
Chronic Obstructive Pulmonary Disease
]

NEIL SCHACHTER, M.D.

BROADWAY BOOKS NEW YORK

A hardcover edition of this book was published in 2003 by
Broadway Books.

PRINTED IN THE UNITED STATES OF AMERICA

BROADWAY BOOKS and its logo, a letter B bisected on the diagonal, are
trademarks of Random House, Inc.

Visit our website at www.broadwaybooks.com

First trade paperback edition published 2004

Book design by Chris Welch
Illustrations by Enid Faltreco and Elizabeth Sample

The Library of Congress has cataloged the hardcover edition as
follows:
Schachter, Neil.
   Life and breath : preventing, treating, and reversing chronic
obstructive pulmonary disease / by Neil Schachter.
      p.   cm.
   Includes bibliographical references and index.
   1. Lungs—Diseases, Obstructive—Popular works. I. Title.
RC776.O3 S347 2003
616.2'4—dc21   2002038368

ISBN 0-7679-1289-6

1   3   5   7   9   10   8   6   4   2

Dedication

In the late 1930s my father, Franz Schachter, was beginning what promised to be a prestigious career as a professor of pathology at the University of Vienna Medical School. When Hitler swept through Eastern Europe, Dad fled Austria to the safety of France. He hired a beautiful, blonde student from the Sorbonne to tutor him in French and began working as a physician in Paris. His security was destroyed again when German troops took over his newly adopted home. He tried to keep a low profile, but was soon rounded up and taken to a detention center at the outskirts of Paris. He was slated to be deported to the work camps in Germany, when he treated and cured a guard of a painful skin problem. In gratitude, the guard allowed my father to escape. He gave Dad a clean overcoat and a German hunting hat and Dad walked out of the prison in the middle of the day. Along with his tutor, who became my mother, he traveled across Europe in an effort to evade capture and reach America. He finally landed in Portugal and in a series of events straight out of the movie *Casablanca,* my parents secured passage to Cuba and then to the United States.

They landed in New York and Dad set up a general practice in the South Bronx. Our first home was a ground floor three-room apartment. We lived in the back bedroom, and his office occupied the front dining and living rooms. Dad loved his patients and they returned the feeling. The South Bronx was and still is a very poor neighborhood and in the days before Medicare and Medicaid, his patients often had no money to pay for health care. When they could not even afford the two dollars he charged for a visit, Dad never billed them, pressing into their hands sample packs of free medication as they left. To show their gratitude, they gave him what they could and our house always was filled with homemade coffee cake, mufflers, preserves, and, for some reason, a seemingly inexhaustible supply of hand-painted ties.

Dad made house calls every night and when I grew old enough, he would take me along. At first I would sit in the car, waiting for him to tell me about the people he had just seen. When I entered my teens, he would take me in to see the patients. One night we went to see a woman with poorly controlled diabetes. She was in pulmonary edema and gasping for breath. To me she looked hours away from death. My dad calmly reached into his black bag, gave her a shot of Mercuhydrin, a diuretic, and helped her swallow a digitalis tablet. The next evening when we returned, the "dying woman" was sitting up in bed, knitting a bright green muffler for her doctor. It was that night I decided to become a doctor, just like my dad.

Dad died just as I was beginning my internship at Bellevue. I still miss him and so do his patients. Several times a year when people see my name on a credit slip or name tag they will say, "Schachter? Are you by any chance related to Dr. Schachter from Avenue St. John?" When they hear he was my father, they tell me another story of his compassion and the care that he gave them and their family. Franz Schachter taught me how to be a better man as well as a better doctor, and it is to his memory that I dedicate this book.

Contents

Medical Disclaimer

This book is not intended to take the place of medical advice from a trained medical professional. Readers are advised to consult their physician or other qualified health professional regarding treatment of their medical problems. Neither the publisher nor the author takes any responsibility for any possible consequences from any treatment, action, or application of medicine, herb, or preparation to any person reading or following the information in this book.

The names and circumstances of the patients have been changed to protect their privacy.

Chapter 1

Introduction

I recognized Maxwell Harris immediately. It had been more than twenty years since I had been an undergraduate in his political science class. On a Columbia campus filled with intellectual all-stars, Maxwell Harris was a legend. He had been an advisor to every President since John Kennedy, and his best-selling books were classics in their field. But it was his personality and style that packed each seat in the large lecture hall. Compelling and articulate, he would sit at the lectern chain-smoking gold-tipped English Ovals. He would smoke each one down to the very tip and then, without taking a break, light the next cigarette with his last puff.

"My wife said she would divorce me if I didn't see a doctor about my cough," he told me as I examined him. "It keeps her up at night and she claims I'm banned from Lincoln Center for drowning out *La Sylphide*," he said with the same dry wit that charmed generations of students. "Can you give me a cough medicine that really works?"

But Professor Harris didn't have just a simple cough and he

would need more than cough syrup. I had to tell my intellectual hero that he had chronic obstructive pulmonary disease or COPD.

He is far from alone. Over the years there has been a relentless rise in the number of cases of COPD throughout the world. In my practice at Mount Sinai Medical Center in New York City, more than 40 percent of my patients now suffer from this debilitating and frequently fatal disease. It is estimated that COPD affects 35 million Americans, but only half are aware that a lingering cough, chronic bronchitis, and shortness of breath are signs of this serious health problem.

> On an international level, COPD affects more than 20 million people in Europe, almost 30 million in Latin America, and a staggering 258 million in Asia.

The Rise of an Equal Opportunity Killer

In the mid-1960s when I was in training at Bellevue Hospital, COPD was seen as a disease of old men. Most of my COPD patients were men in their sixties who had lived and played hard. Heavy drinkers with nicotine-stained fingers, they rattled windows with their coughs, keeping other patients up at night. One day I was on rounds with Dr. John McClement, the grand old man of chest medicine. In the 1920s, tuberculosis was arguably the leading public health problem in large cities in the United States. Director of the chest service at Bellevue, Dr. McClement was one of the people credited for bringing this once fatal and epidemic disease under control in New York City. That particular morning there had been more than the usual number of people with COPD admitted to the floor and there was some confusion about the patients. In their blue-and-white hospital gowns, and with their unshaven faces covered with oxygen masks, the four older men looked almost identical. "Maybe we should just number them," I joked with the insensitivity of a very young doctor.

Dr. McClement just nudged me with his elbow. "See those young women at the nursing station?" he asked, pointing to a group of nurses lighting up cigarettes with their morning coffee. "In twenty years, they too will be your patients," he predicted.

Unfortunately, he was right. Over the past two decades, I have seen a sharp rise in the number of people affected with COPD. No longer a disease of aged roués, my COPD patients include dancers, ambassadors, writers, teachers, and reporters. Even more troubling has been the startling increase in the number of women with COPD. Figures from The National Center for Health Statistics report that the rate of COPD has risen in women 100 percent since 1992.

Watching the Women

Dr. McClement's prediction was especially ominous because of the importance that epidemiologists place on disease incidence in women. Epidemiology is the study of patterns of disease. Who they are and where people become ill provides critical clues that can help us prevent and cure illness. In any situation, there can be many possible causes of disease and one of the first clues is: "Look at the women."

In the past, men have been exposed to a greater number of

environmental and other risk factors. They have until recently tended to drink more, smoke more, drive faster, use more illicit drugs, work in more dangerous environments, have a higher risk of heart disease, and been more likely to carry weapons. Teasing out which of these factors is affecting death and disease rates is complex and subject to partisan debate. For example, for decades it was the presence of these multiple factors that helped cigarette companies successfully avoid blame for tobacco-related health issues.

For a better picture of the cause and incidence of an illness, we frequently look at the health status of women. Historically, we have learned that a rise in the number of women affected is a sign that a disease is spreading more rapidly. During my years at Bellevue, I can remember only a handful of women who were diagnosed with COPD. In the years that have followed, Dr. McClement's prediction has slowly but steadily come true. Today almost half of the people with COPD are women, a sign of equality no one ever wanted to see.

I am particularly frustrated that by the time both men and women come to my office, many have had COPD for five to ten years. During that time, their lungs have suffered serious and irreversible damage. There is so little awareness of COPD that it often takes a major health crisis to get them the health care they need. It is especially troubling because we have learned so much about the underlying dynamics of the body's airways and have translated this knowledge into effective care strategies. We have developed a wide range of medications that control symptoms and may slow loss of lung function. We have identified pollutants in our environment and developed filters to clean our homes and offices. Now we have even identified the role of diet and the importance of antioxidants for pulmonary health.

This book, *Life and Breath*, allows me an incredible opportunity to alert you to potentially serious health problems while there is still time to take the necessary steps to relieve symptoms and prevent further damage. In addition to alerting people who already have COPD, I am equally concerned about reaching the 95 million current and former smokers in America who are at increased risk for developing COPD. *Life and Breath* will offer step-by-step practical programs for diet, exercise, medical care, and environmental protection that will yield long-term protective and preventive measures.

Life and Breath is particularly important for the 26 million Americans with asthma. This is the first book to explain how asthma, once seen as a separate disease, can lead to COPD, even in people who have never smoked cigarettes. This book will offer simple yet effective advice to prevent the development of chronic irreversible pulmonary symptoms in asthmatics.

What Is COPD?

COPD occurs when airflow is reduced through the lungs due to the development, either singly or in combination, of chronic bronchitis and emphysema. Chronic bronchitis is defined as a chronic "wet" cough that occurs for months at a time, two years in a row. Emphysema is an abnormal permanent enlargement of the air sacs (called alveoli) in the lungs. This damage eventually causes severe shortness of breath and wheezing.

Historically, asthma was considered a separate disorder from these. Asthma was regarded as an acute but reversible problem, primarily seen in younger patients and linked to allergies. Once the asthma attack passed, lung function was felt to return to normal. By contrast, COPD was considered a chronic, progressive disease, usually occurring after age fifty and closely linked to cigarette smoking. In recent years, we have changed our perceptions and now see asthma as part of COPD. Along with my pulmonary colleagues, I began to see a widespread pattern among asthmatics suggesting that they were developing true irreversible pulmonary constriction characteristic of COPD. While asthma was supposed to disappear between attacks, we saw people developing the chronic shortness of breath once thought to be characteristic of emphysema and chronic bronchitis. Our observations were backed up with laboratory tests. We found that people with asthma were showing the same permanent decline in lung function normally seen in classic COPD patients. It is now clear that asthma is a true member of the COPD family. In fact, it is not uncommon for a patient to have a combination of asthma, bronchitis, and emphysema.

These findings are not just of academic interest but have a critical impact on health care. When asthma and COPD overlap, we need to take a different approach to managing symptoms and preventing permanent lung damage. Although the symptoms can be very similar, the underlying cellular and biochemical changes are different and it is important to adjust your care to take these differences into consideration. For example, "asthmatic COPD" often has a strong allergic component that needs to be treated for maximum symptom control.

Could I Get COPD?

To measure personal COPD risk, ask yourself these questions:

- Did you start smoking as a teenager?
- Did you grow up in a household where one or more of your parents smoked?
- Do you now smoke at least ten cigarettes a day? Did you do so in the past?
- Have you ever been told that you have asthma?
- Do other members of your family have allergies?
- Do you have allergies?
- Does anyone in your close family have asthma?
- Did you get frequent colds as a child?
- As an adult, do colds tend to develop into a lingering cough?
- Do you quickly get out of breath when you run?
- Do you become short of breath when you climb a flight of stairs?
- Does your chest feel tight in cold weather?
- Do you live or work near electrical power plants or other smokestack industries?
- Do you live or work in areas with heavy automobile traffic?
- Do you work in a job where the air quality is monitored by the Occupational Safety and Health Administration (OSHA) (e.g., cotton mill, bakery, ironworks, furniture plant, toll booth)?

If you answered yes to at least three or four of these questions, you should consider yourself at high risk for COPD. In the chapters that follow, I will give you the information you need to protect your lungs and your health.

In Chapter Two, "The Healthy Lung," I will define the different parts of the pulmonary system and the changes that can occur with COPD. I have found that a basic understanding of the design and function of the lungs is critical for my patients to understand how to protect and care for their health. For example, most people with COPD will be given several types of inhalers. One inhaler often contains an anti-inflammatory spray that acts to prevent long-term damage to lung structure. This one should be used every day, whether or not you have symptoms, to stop problems before they happen. A second type of inhaler is known as rescue medication that acts immediately to deal with sudden symptoms such as shortness of breath. Being able to visualize how each type of medication works in the lungs helps people know which one to use at the right time.

Chapter Three explores the signs and symptoms of different types of lung disease. It will probably be a shock to some readers to realize that the so-called smoker's cough is frequently a sign of COPD, not just a minor annoyance. Although your blood tests and X rays can be normal, that nagging cough may be the pulmonary equivalent of the flashing red light on the dashboard that tells you to see a mechanic immediately. This chapter describes the problems and stages of each type of COPD. It explains how changes in the lungs relate to the symptoms and what that means in terms of treatment.

Chapter Four, "The Causes of COPD," analyzes how lifestyle, the environment, and physiological factors are linked to COPD. It looks at heredity, allergies, stress, and air pollution, and assesses their impact on the pulmonary system. To help prevent problems, I will emphasize the difference between factors that cause COPD and those that simply trigger symptoms.

Chapter Five, "The Complete Chest Workup," takes you through a complete lung exam. It begins with a look at your medical history and explains what your answers are telling you and your physician about your health. The chapter continues with a map of the physical examination. From head to toe, I'll tell you what your doctor is looking for and the implications of the findings. The chapter closes with an in-depth analysis of pulmonary function tests that measure the critical strengths and weaknesses of your lungs.

I'm fairly certain that you can tell your last blood pressure reading and your cholesterol level, but may have never heard of lung function tests such as forced vital capacity or residual volume. I want you to understand the values of these tests because they can give us an accurate evaluation of pulmonary health as well as measure the effectiveness of your treatment program.

If you have pulmonary problems, Chapter Six, "Eat Right, Breathe Easy," may change the way you cook and eat. This chapter explores the importance of diet in asthma and COPD. Large-scale studies have now shown that people who have high levels of antioxidants in their blood have lower incidence of asthma and emphysema. Interestingly, even when COPD has developed in the countries with higher intakes of fruits and vegetables, the disease has been less severe and the death rates were lower. A study presented at a recent meeting of the American Thoracic Society reported that a single apple a day cut the risk of COPD by more than 50 percent.

Chapter Six discusses why certain foods offer pulmonary protection and the unsatisfactory results when we tried to duplicate these findings with just vitamin supplements. In this chapter, I will explain how to use the results of these scientific studies in planning pulmonary protective meals. In addition to looking at foods that protect lung function, I'm going to examine the common minerals that can increase shortness of breath.

Chapter Six also reviews the importance of weight control in asthma. As a clinician, I have observed that when asthmatic patients gain weight, their symptoms become more severe. A paper published in the *Archives of Internal Medicine* backed up these observations. In a study of 86,000 nurses, researchers from Harvard found that obese women were three times more likely to develop asthma than their thinner colleagues. Doctors suggest that the extra weight makes the body work harder or may reduce available lung volume. I will provide a diet and exercise program that will help you lose weight as well as offer nutrients that reduce oxidative stress in the lungs.

Exercise is at least as important as nutrition for respiratory health. Chapter Seven, "The Pulmonary Protective Workout," will describe how COPD limits the flow of oxygen into the lungs and shows how exercise can improve oxygen delivery throughout the body. This chapter outlines the heart and lung testing that must be done in order to design an exercise program that takes into account your physical status and exercise needs. It evaluates the three different types of exercise and how each type can assist breathing. I'll illustrate how even a daily brisk walk can improve pulmonary status, offer weight-training exercises to increase oxygen delivery, and demonstrate stretching exercises to relieve shortness of breath.

Cigarette smoking is the 800-pound gorilla in my office. We all know it's there, but it is very difficult to get rid of. No book on COPD would be complete without a chapter that explores the best ways to quit. Chapter Eight, "It's Never Too Late to Quit," begins with an exploration of the psychology and physiology of smoking addiction. *Life and Breath* never condemns or scolds smokers. People who are struggling with smoking are NOT stupid, self-destructive, lazy, or unmotivated. I want every smoker to understand that nicotine in their cigarettes is every bit as addictive as alcohol or cocaine. The chapter evaluates the different antismoking drugs and explains the best way to use them. In closing, I'll discuss the best ways to use alternative therapies such as hypnosis and acupuncture in combination with antismoking medications.

Chapter Nine, "Treatment Strategies for Asthma and COPD," is focused on the medical options and treatment choices that can potentially control symptoms and reverse lung damage. New studies and research have provided greater insight into the causes and progression of COPD. These discoveries have allowed us to develop a wide range of treatment strategies that offer help at every stage of the disease.

There are five different categories of treatment that either singly or in combination relieve symptoms and protect lung function. I'll pinpoint how each class of drugs works, the right way to use them, and their potential side effects. This chapter also explores the importance of preventing chronic inflammation, in order to avoid the development of irreversible damage to the airways, as well as a review of the preventive strategies such as vaccines, antibiotics, and the latest antiviral agents. The chapter closes with a look at alternative therapies such as biofeedback, acupuncture, and meditation, explaining how to incorporate them into your treatment plan.

Chapter Ten, "The Healthy Home," looks at the environmental issues in your home. In this chapter, I will offer step-by-step practical advice to improve air quality in every aspect of your daily lives. I will take you on a walking tour of your home, pointing out irritants and triggers. For example, I'll help you find sources of mold-producing moisture, help you reduce allergens from pets, and explain how to choose the most effective air filters and cleaning products.

Chapter Eleven, "Healthy Lungs at Work and at Play," examines the pulmonary problems that you can experience at work and at play. It looks at ways to clean up your work environment, explores healthy travel strategies, and deals with irritants that we use in hobbies and crafts. For example, it looks at the breathing problems you may encounter on a plane and how to control them.

Life and Breath will close with a question and answer section that draws on over twenty-five years of experience in pulmonary medicine. From the value of moving to another climate to the use of yoga to control asthma, this chapter takes a sensitive look at the personal and social problems that can be part of COPD.

Who Needs This Book?

COPD is arguably the most underdiagnosed and undertreated health problem in the United States. The American Thoracic Society estimates that only half of the 35 million Americans with COPD are aware that their lingering cough or shortness of breath is a symptom of a serious, chronic illness. A new study from Johns Hopkins indicates that this estimate may have been much too low. This study recently examined data from 150 patients admitted over a six-month period. In this group, fully one quarter had pulmonary problems, but only 35 percent of these respiratory patients were correctly diagnosed.

It is my hope that *Life and Breath* will raise awareness of COPD in both doctors and patients. It is my firm belief that early, accurate diagnosis of your pulmonary problems will help you live a longer and healthier life.

Chapter 2

The Healthy Lung

If you like soup and live in southern Connecticut, then you probably know my patient Marisa. At her narrow, cozy restaurant, she makes two different types of delicious soup each day and serves them with a slice of her equally famous oatmeal bread. An asthma sufferer, Marisa would get confused about how and when to use the different types of pills and sprays. After two bad (and unnecessary) asthmatic attacks, I tried a different approach. We sat down together with an anatomy book and I explained the function of each part of the respiratory system and how these parts were affected by the medications. The anatomy lesson worked better than I could have ever imagined. Marisa now understood the principles behind each drug and knew exactly how and when to treat her symptoms. I also learned an important lesson that day: not to underestimate the intelligence of my patients.

A Marvel of Design

The lungs basically have three main jobs—take in air, distribute oxygen, and remove carbon dioxide. Yet, to accomplish these straightforward tasks, they need a remarkably complex physiological system to exchange gases connected to a mechanical marvel of design. Understanding the design and function of the pulmonary system is the basis for preventing and reversing pulmonary problems.

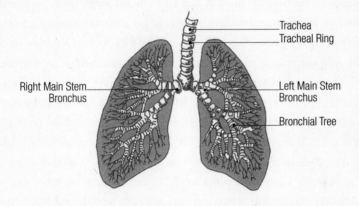

The primary structures of the pulmonary system are the lungs, trachea, and bronchial tree.

The job of respiration starts at the trachea, the large tube in the center of your throat. The trachea is basically composed of soft tissue that is held open by a scaffold of cartilage rings that encircle the trachea like horseshoes around a bar. This support system is soft enough to be flexible, but strong enough to hold the airways open. The trachea begins at the voice box or

Adam's apple, continues through the opening in the top of the chest, and goes into the chest about halfway down the length of your breastbone (sternum).

At that point, the trachea divides in two and changes its name. It is now known as the bronchi and branches into two divisions. There is a right main stem bronchus that goes into the right lung, and a left main stem bronchus that goes into the left lung. Each lung is formed into lobes, with three lobes on the right side and two lobes on the left. They correspond to the first and second division of the trachea after the branching begins. The first division is the right main stem bronchus and the left main stem bronchus, which go into the right and left lung, respectively. The right main stem bronchus divides into three branches, an upper, middle, and lower division, while the left main stem divides into an upper and lower division. These branchings correspond to the lobes of the lungs. Each lobe is separated anatomically by the infoldings of the surface coating of the lungs that is the pleura. We are normally unaware of the pleura until there is an inflammation or infection of that tissue, a condition known as pleurisy. It causes a characteristic sharp pain that can be felt when sitting completely still, and becomes even worse when coughing, talking, taking a deep breath, walking, or moving around.

The fact that the lungs are divided into separate lobes has important medical consequences. It helps to keep tumors and infections localized, preventing destruction of the entire organ. Lung surgeons, working to remove the smallest amount of tissue possible, try to limit the operation to just one lobe to preserve maximum function.

The bronchi within the lobes continue to divide. If we

consider each division as one level, then, on average, the bronchial tree, as it is known, divides twenty-three times. That may not seem like a lot, until you consider that it represents an exponential number, 2^{23} branches. When you get to that kind of number, you're talking about millions and millions of tiny airways. By the time you get to the level of the twenty-third division, the individual tiny airways are far less than one millimeter in diameter. But if you add up all of the cross-sectional areas of these airways, as well as the area of the membrane that covers them, then the surface area of this part of the lung is greater than that of a tennis court. That's pretty amazing when you consider that the original cross-sectional area of the trachea (the site of the first division) was only about the size of a Coke bottle cap.

The large surface area is one of the reasons the lungs can sustain so much damage before breathing is compromised. The good news is that an otherwise healthy person can actually

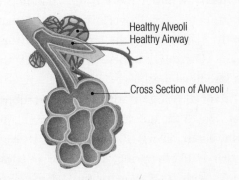

Healthy Alveoli
Healthy Airway

Cross Section of Alveoli

Healthy, intact alveoli budding off a clear, open airway

survive with the equivalent of only one lung. The bad news is that this large lung reserve allows us to smoke cigarettes for years without consciously suffering from the damage that is occurring.

At about the seventeenth division, we begin to notice out-pouchings (little sacs) called alveoli. Each alveolus is essentially one cell thick. This very thin cell separates the inner part of the alveolus from the tiny capillary blood vessels that coat them. It is at this level that gases are exchanged. In other words, the oxygen from the air we breathe diffuses through the walls of both the alveolus and the capillary, where it combines with hemoglobin to be transported to the rest of the body. Additionally, carbon dioxide (which is the end product of all metabolism that is going on in your body) is now transferred from the blood to the alveoli, from which it can be eliminated. As you exhale, the air that is now rich in carbon dioxide and poor in oxygen is exhaled.

The alveoli are surrounded by a mesh network of collagen and elastin fibers. Without the elastin scaffolding to maintain normal structure, the alveoli overinflate and are unable to function efficiently. Elastin allows the lungs to maintain their structural integrity. Damage to these fibers causes the lungs to enlarge and lose flexibility.

It is important to recognize that the lung is subjected to two elastic forces. One is the pull inward of its own elastic structural elements, the elastin fibers. The other pull is from the bony chest wall that is like a spring, which expands outward and pulls the lungs with it. If most of the "elastic" bands (elastin fibers) that are pulling the lung inward are "cut," as they are in emphysema, the lung overexpands and becomes very large.

That is a very inefficient position for breathing to occur. When the lungs expand outward, your diaphragm drops down to a position that no longer allows you to move air in and out comfortably.

From Macro to Micro

Now that we've covered the large structures of the pulmonary system, I want to explore with you the cellular aspects of the lung. The upper airway composed of the trachea and the main bronchi are lined by a mucous membrane. The surface of this mucous membrane is made up of cells that have a very specific look to them. The technical term for these cells is pseudostratified columnar epithelium. What that means in English is that these are very long, tall cells and they grow up from a surface that is composed of connective tissue called the basement membrane. These pseudocolumnar cells have two major functions. A majority of them have tiny cilia, little hairs on the inside surface of the airway. They move back and forth, like wheat in a field being blown by the wind. They have a constant motion, flowing slowly in one direction and quickly in another. The cilia are covered with a coat of mucus that acts much like flypaper for the lungs, attracting dirt and bacteria that we breathe in. The little hairs allow the mucus to move up toward the mouth, where you can spit it out or swallow it so it's no longer a danger to your lungs.

Additional mucus is produced by tiny glands originating underneath the submucosal layer of the airway. In addition to these glands, this tissue contains blood vessels, smooth muscle, and supporting collagen. It is this muscle that allows the airways to either contract or relax. In other words, this muscle allows the airways to become narrow and tight or relaxed and open.

We don't exactly understand why these muscles are there. We suspect that, for the most part, they are intended to stabilize the airways to make sure they remain open. When you take in a breath, you want the airways to expand, so the muscles have to relax a bit. When you breathe out, you want the airways to squeeze a little bit to help the air be emptied and so they contract slightly. When needed, you use these muscles to help you when you cough. But they are probably best known by the fact that they can suddenly become constricted. They overreact and are very sensitive to all sorts of stimuli, particularly in people with asthma or bronchitis. One of the main problems with asthma is that these muscles overreact to simple, everyday irritant factors such as cold air or perfume. The normal balancing mechanisms that keep them at the right length no longer apply. Very suddenly, they can contract and close off the airways.

The Cellular Biology of the Lung

As you move down to the very smallest airways, the cartilage that began as rings in the trachea now covers less and less of the airway. It appears as little patches that become increasingly scarce as the bronchi become smaller and smaller. By the time you get down to the smallest airways, there is no more cartilage. At this point, the pseudocolumnar epithelial cells begin to flatten and their cilia disappear. Goblet cells disappear and other cells appear and develop specialized roles.

There are two types of important cells to recognize in these tiny airways. Type I cells are there for support, covering most of the surface of the smaller airways and alveoli. It is through these very tiny flat cells that oxygen and carbon dioxide move easily. There are also Type II cells, which produce a substance called surfactant that helps reduce the surface tension on the alveoli to keep them from collapsing in on themselves. In premature babies, these Type II cells are not fully mature, and the surfactant is either not completely functional or not formed at all. For this reason, babies can develop what is known as hyaline membrane disease, or respiratory distress syndrome of the newborn. This problem occurs because the air-exchanging air sacs, the alveoli, collapse and cannot transport oxygen into the bloodstream, nor can they help get rid of carbon dioxide.

In the 1960s, President and Mrs. Kennedy lost a premature baby to hyaline membrane disease. Since that time, we've made quite a bit of progress in understanding this problem. We now understand how to use artificial ventilation while babies' lungs mature enough to produce this essential surfactant.

We have also developed a therapeutic version of surfactant that can be injected into these very tiny lungs and can help prevent or at least reduce the time they remain collapsed. We also better understand some of the hormonal reasons why the lungs do not mature when babies are born prematurely, and we can give some of them hormones to accelerate the development of the surfactants so that these infants recover more quickly.

The Architecture of the Pulmonary System

The physiological and cellular aspects of the respiratory system are just one part of the breathing process. The mechanical act of breathing plays an equally important role in pulmonary health and disease.

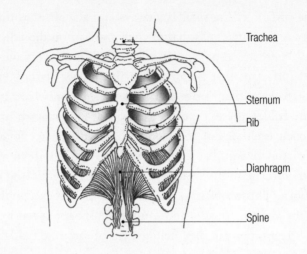

Trachea

Sternum

Rib

Diaphragm

Spine

The bony frame of the thorax houses and protects the
soft tissue of the airways.

The pulmonary system is a complex design of different muscles and bony structures. A pyramid-shaped configuration, the chest starts at the thoracic outlet, which is where the neck comes out of the chest, and follows the rib cage down to the diaphragm. It is bounded on the sides and back by the ribs, which are attached to the vertebrae of the spine in the back, and in front by the sternum or breastbone. These bones, connected to muscles and ligaments, allow us to breathe in a rhythmic way. How we breathe depends on what we're doing. When we're at rest, the diaphragm is designed to be the principal muscle of breathing. Attached to the bottom of the rib cage, its contractions brings the lungs down, enlarging them, and, by so doing, draws air into the airways.

When the diaphragm relaxes, the lungs, propelled by their elastic tissue, move upward. This compresses them and air is forced out of the lungs. At rest we normally repeat this motion twelve to sixteen times a minute, every day of our lives. Called resting ventilation, it supplies the air you need when you're not performing any exercise or making additional efforts. When you become more active and start walking around or doing housework, more parts of the thorax come into play. These are the times you need more air moving in and out of your lungs, in order to deliver oxygen for energy and remove waste carbon dioxide. For a healthy person, this happens during such activities as yardwork, exercise, or dancing. For someone with pulmonary problems, the need for additional ventilation can even occur in a situation where you are essentially at rest.

To obtain the additionally needed air, you have to move the rest of your chest. You will do this with two different motions. The first is the so-called "pail handle" motion. The ribs can rotate up and down, just like the handle of a pail. When you move the rib cage upward, you increase the volume of the chest, because by pulling up, the ribs pivot upward and outward. This increases the volume within the chest and, just like a bellows, draws air into the lungs. When the "handles of the pail" move down as you relax, the volume inside the chest decreases, and air is pushed out.

The third way to move air in and out of the chest is actually to move the entire thorax, the chest wall and bony structure, up and down. This is accomplished through a system of muscles in the neck that are attached to your collarbone and the upper ribs. When these muscles contract, they pull up the top of the chest wall. This increases the volume of the chest, increasing the amount of air that can be drawn in. By relaxing these muscles, you breathe out.

Known as accessory muscles of respiration, these muscles between the ribs and the neck tend to tire very easily. These muscles were never meant to do breathing for any length of time. People without pulmonary problems use accessory muscles to increase breathing during exertion. But when the lungs are struggling, such as during an asthmatic attack or continuously in severe chronic lung disease, these muscles are called upon to work far beyond their capacity. In Chapter Seven, we're going to look at ways to stretch out these muscles to improve endurance, and avoid cramping and exhaustion.

Putting Theory into Practice

Like my patient Marisa, you now have a good picture of the major parts of the respiratory system and some of their functions. We looked at the tissues, the skeletal system, the muscles, and special structures like alveoli and bronchi that are needed to breathe. But it is how they work together that provides insight into the link between structure and function, and health and disease.

There are actually five separate but related functions of the pulmonary system and we measure them to judge how well (or how poorly) the lungs are working.

Static Lung Function: This is just a simple way of measuring lung size. This is important to evaluate because in disease the lungs may change size or may not be able to expand fully so that the amount of air that you can move in and out may be diminished.

When we are children, the lungs are very small. As we become adults, the lungs grow with us. When we grow older, the lungs naturally diminish in size. We expect that the lungs of an eighty-year-old person to be smaller than the corresponding lungs of a twenty-year-old person, taking into account various body characteristics, such as height, weight, sex, and race.

Vital Capacity: The maximum volume of air that can be moved in and out of the lung with slow breathing is known as the *vital capacity* or *VC*. It is six or seven times larger than the amount of air that we move in and out of the lung when we breathe at rest. This volume of breath taken at rest is known as the *tidal volume*. The extra volume that we have available to us (when more oxygen is required by the body so that it can function at higher levels) is known as the *inspiratory* and *expiratory reserve volumes*. This reserve is important to us when we want to increase the level of our activity, such as with exercise.

Residual Volume: There always exists in the lung a volume of air that cannot be exhaled, no matter how hard we try. This volume is known as the *residual volume (RV)* and in a sense prevents our lungs from collapsing. This would be a very unhealthy state of affairs because a collapsed lung is difficult to reinflate. In obstructive lung disease like COPD, the *residual volume* increases as a result of air trapping and the loss of the lung's normal elastic recoil. Frequently, this is accompanied by a loss in *vital capacity*.

Restrictive lung diseases limit our ability to use our full *vital capacity*. What happens in these diseases can be visualized by the scenario of having someone tie a rope around your chest and pull on the ends. This restriction limits your ability to take in a deep breath. The measurements of vital capacity under these circumstances are smaller.

Dynamic Lung Function: This measures how efficiently

the lungs work when air moves rapidly through the airways. We breathe by moving the diaphragm and the chest wall so that air can be propelled in and out of the lung through the airways, at a rate dictated by our metabolic needs. Different situations, either singly or in combination, can affect *dynamic lung function*. In chronic bronchitis, airflow can be compromised by mucus plugs in the airways. In asthma attacks, spasms that narrow airways will impede airflow. In people with emphysema, the airways become flabby and collapse, limiting airflow. It is possible to have both or several of these problems simultaneously.

Exchange/Diffusion Functions: The primary job of the respiratory system is to deliver oxygen and remove carbon dioxide to and from the blood. Measuring the *gas exchange/diffusion functions* tells us how efficiently oxygen and other gases are transported to and from the alveolus into the blood of the capillaries. This function of gas exchange depends on how well the alveoli are receiving air, the thickness of the lung tissue between the alveolus and the capillary, the amount of blood circulating in the capillaries, and the ability of the lungs to match ventilation with circulation.

Diffusion problems occur in a number of different pulmonary diseases. In emphysema, the circulation of blood through the capillaries surrounding the alveoli is significantly reduced, leading to a decrease in diffusion. Pulmonary fibrosis causes scar tissue to form in the lungs, thickening the barrier between the alveoli and capillary. In pulmonary edema, where heart failure causes fluid to build up in the lungs, the alveoli become flooded and air has great difficulty diffusing into the capillaries.

Biochemical Functions: Just like the liver or the pancreas, the lung has *biochemical functions* producing hormones and other chemical substances that help the body function normally. For example, the lungs are the site of an enzyme called angiotensin-converting enzyme (ACE), which is critical for the regulation of blood pressure.

Because so much blood travels through the pulmonary system, the lungs act as a filter of toxic agents and can also transform and inactivate biological compounds.

The lungs are at the interface of the outside environment (the air) and the inner environment of the bloodstream. As such, the lungs must protect the inner environment against everything that we inhale. For example, dust particles, gases, fumes, bacteria, and viruses must be inactivated or removed before they can damage not only the lung but the body in general. Fortunately, the lungs can accomplish this in several ways. We've seen how the airways are covered with a thick sticky mucus that traps particles and soluble agents and how these can be expelled. In some rare hereditary disorders, the cilia that line the airways are dysfunctional and this can lead to repeated lung infections. This disease is often accompanied in men by sterility because the same mechanism which keeps cilia beating also powers the tail of the sperm cells.

Immunologic Functions: The airways and the alveoli also have within them immunologic cells, usually white blood cells, that act to engulf and destroy inhaled foreign materials, such as dust particles, bacteria, or viruses that are inhaled as we breathe. We can measure this *immunologic function* by looking at the type and number of white blood cells in the airways. For example, in allergic asthma, we will expect to find large numbers of the white blood cell known as the eosinophil. In bronchitis, we find a different type of white blood cell, called neutrophils. These observations can help us pinpoint a diagnosis where lung problems have similar symptoms.

Knowing the parts of the lung and how they function, we can now begin to understand the different types of chronic lung diseases, and how they affect the pulmonary system.

Chapter 3

What Is COPD?

I think of COPD as the "orphan disease" that affects 35 million Americans. Although chronic obstructive pulmonary disease is the fourth-leading cause of death in the United States, most people have not heard of this debilitating and sometimes fatal disease. European respiratory and pulmonary experts recently predicted that by the year 2020 COPD will be the third-most deadly disease in the world. A survey that looked at the incidence and demographics of COPD in North America and Europe found a great deal of ignorance and misinformation about the disease. Most people, including physicians, saw COPD as a problem of older men. In fact, 44 percent of patients with COPD are women, and over half of all patients are between the ages of forty-five and sixty-four. Even more troubling, one out of four patients with pulmonary problems didn't believe that their physicians could do anything to relieve their symptoms.

Lack of awareness means that diagnosis and treatment often occur after the disease had gone unchecked for years. During this time, lung and airway anatomy undergoes an unhealthy process known as remodeling, a progressive alteration in lung anatomy and architecture that impairs pulmonary function.

Pulmonary remodeling goes to the very heart of the goals of this book. It is my belief that preventive and early treatment strategies can stop or limit the debilitating irreversible effects of remodeling. In order to understand what this means in terms of your respiratory health, it is important to understand the different forms of COPD.

Chronic Bronchitis—When a Cough Is More Than a Cough

The symptom, often known as smoker's cough, is that annoying "wet" cough that never seems to go away. It keeps you up at night. It wakes you up in the morning and disrupts plays and concerts for everyone else. It is so much a part of many people's day that most are unaware they are coughing.

I remember two women who came to my office for examination. As I sat at my desk, I could hear a rattling cough from the very full waiting room. Even my nurse, who has heard more than her share of coughs, winced at the sound. As I was examining my next patient, a young pregnant woman with asthma, I asked my nurse to see if the "cougher" could be seen sooner rather than later so that I could schedule an X ray for that afternoon. "Oh!" said my patient, laughing. "That's my Aunt Sylvia. She doesn't have an appointment. Aunt Sylvia drove me so I wouldn't have to go on the subway. She always has that cough," she assured me. "It's been going on for years." When I finished my examination of the expectant mother, I went to the waiting room to bring in Aunt Sylvia. I convinced her to schedule an appointment, and as I suspected, she had the most common form of COPD, chronic bronchitis.

We are not meant to cough continuously. A cough is the body's reaction to an irritant in the airways. This irritation provokes excessive mucus that builds up and irritates and blocks the airways. Chronic bronchitis is diagnosed by a history of coughing and phlegm. We define chronic bronchitis as an illness in which a patient admits that they've had a productive cough for several months a year for at least two years in a row. There is usually very little visible on X rays. Sometimes the lungs have what we call a "dirty" appearance, because airway walls and the tissues between the air sacs have become thickened and inflamed. On an X ray, there is an excess of linear markings on the film and the airways appear swollen.

When the bronchial tree has been irritated for a long time, the lining becomes thickened and inflamed. As a result, it

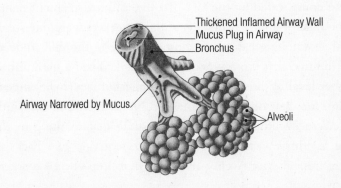

With chronic bronchitis, the airways are narrowed by swelling and inflammation as well as blocked with mucus.

becomes harder to breathe. Mucus accumulation becomes a fertile place for bacterial growth. When this occurs, chronic bronchitis can be complicated by an acute exacerbation or infection that may include fever, a worsening cough, and an increase in shortness of breath.

Chronic bronchitis affects 5 percent of Americans or 15 million people. The overwhelming cause of this disease in cigarette smoking. In addition, people who work in industries with unhealthy levels of fumes and dust, like mining and metalwork, are also prone to develop signs and symptoms of chronic bronchitis.

If you are exposed to high levels of pollution in your work and you are a smoker, the prevalence and the severity of chronic bronchitis will be far more pronounced. While I was at Yale University, I was involved in epidemiological studies with mill workers in South Carolina. We were looking to demonstrate the impact on breathing of the high levels of cotton dust that would cloud the air where people worked. Our studies were complicated by the fact that the mill management maintained that the lung problems of their workers were due solely to their smoking habits, not dust exposure in the mill. Indeed, we did find that those workers who smoked had a significantly higher level of disease, and this complicated securing compensation for their occupational injury. Nevertheless, in this study we were eventually able to demonstrate that working in the mill for thirty years was equivalent to smoking two packs of cigarettes a day for twenty-five years in its impact on a worker's lungs.

Emphysema—An Insidious Disease

Emphysema, one of the most serious forms of COPD, is characterized by the destruction of alveoli, those little grapelike sacs at the end of the branching bronchial tree. It is here that oxygen first enters the bloodstream and carbon dioxide is removed from the blood. If these alveoli are damaged, then the very basis for breathing is compromised.

In emphysema, the alveoli become overinflated and develop large holes in their walls. After a while, rather than looking like a small compact bunch of grapes, the alveoli look like a piece of old lace. The characteristic symptom of emphysema is extreme shortness of breath, even at rest. There may also be dry cough and quite a bit of fatigue because the body is working so hard to maintain adequate ventilation and oxygen levels.

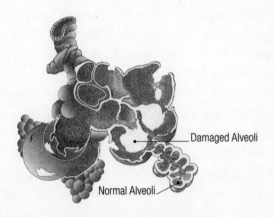

Damaged Alveoli

Normal Alveoli

With emphysema, the alveoli are enlarged and torn, creating large nonfunctional air spaces.

The health and function of the alveoli depend greatly on the elastin fibers that surround them. The body has a natural defense system for protecting these fibers. When threatened by bacteria or toxic chemicals, such as those found in smoke, the body sends out white blood cells called neutrophils to gobble up the offending elements. Neutrophils contain elastase, an enzyme which also eats up damaged elastin fibers, kind of an in-house cleanup system. Elastase is a member of a more generic brand of enzymes that degrade proteins, known as proteases.

Normally, there is a checks-and-balance system in the body with antiprotease molecules being formed to inhibit protease molecules from doing too much damage to healthy tissue. In the lung, the antielastase that is formed prevents excess destruction from elastase. Under healthy conditions, the balance between the elastase/antielastase system protects the lung from infection and foreign elements while preventing overdestruction of elastin fibers. Unfortunately, cigarette smoke destroys this critical balance. The toxins in the smoke attract the rush of neutrophils to the air sacs, provoking the uninhibited release of elastase. At the same time, smoke itself inhibits the production and activity of the antiprotease system.

As a result, the damage from elastase in the neutrophils is unchecked. Over time, alveolar tissue is eaten away until it is destroyed beyond all recognition. As these sacs are destroyed, they are unable to supply oxygen to the bloodstream. In addition, the lungs lose their ability to expand and contract easily. They become overinflated, making it difficult to exhale.

Emphysema progresses slowly and insidiously and most people only become aware of their problem in their fifties or sixties. Many of my patients experience shortness of breath for years before seeking help, attributing their symptoms to pollution or advancing age. By the time they come to me, they may find it difficult to walk a block or to make their bed. As time passes, lung function continues to decline. When a cold or flu develops, emphysema symptoms can suddenly become increasingly severe. Called an acute exacerbation, these attacks produce symptoms of increasing shortness of breath and sometimes fever. Often these acute periods require short hospital stays to avoid respiratory failure. Once stabilized with antibiotics, bronchodilators, anti-inflammatories, and supplemental oxygen, patients usually feel better and can be discharged after a few days. But the underlying problem remains—and must be dealt with.

Looking at the Numbers

It is estimated that 2 million people in the United States have emphysema. While the overwhelming majority develop the problem as a consequence of years of heavy smoking, up to 5 percent suffer from a hereditary form of the disease known as alpha-1 antitrypsin deficiency.

This inherited form of emphysema is caused by the lack of the antiprotease that prevents elastase overdestruction. The symptoms are very similar to traditional emphysema, but appear when an individual is in his or her thirties or forties. If someone with alpha-1 antitrypsin is a smoker, the disease can appear even earlier and in a more severe form. If that person never smokes, the symptoms of lung disease usually appear far later and may not appear at all. In other words, even if you have the underlying, inherited tendency to emphysema but you don't smoke, you may not get sick.

Unlike chronic bronchitis, the diagnosis of emphysema is

based more on laboratory tests than on simply the patient's history and symptoms. When the chief complaint is shortness of breath, we need to look further.

Shortness of breath can occur as a result of a number of problems, including anemia and many different types of heart disease. To nail down a diagnosis, we need to look at pulmonary function tests, X rays, and even CAT scans. On an X ray, people with emphysema have very large lungs, not only because air is trapped in them but because the elastin fibers have been destroyed as well. The chest wall, which is normally pulled inward by the lungs' elastic properties, now overwhelms the lung's elasticity and pulls the lung outward to a larger volume.

CAT scans can also be a very helpful tool for diagnosing emphysema. When reading a CAT scan, the blacker something is, the thinner it is; the whiter it is, the thicker it is. The thickest structures in your chest are the bones. On a CAT scan, you can see the ribs as stark white. The heart, which is mainly tissue and fluid, comes out a more translucent shade of white. On a CAT scan of healthy lungs, the tissue has a white hazy quality. The healthy lung, which is mainly composed of tiny little air sacs, appears grayish white. When there is emphysema present, the CAT scan shows large black areas. Where there once was healthy lung tissue, it is now just air.

It is very common to have both chronic bronchitis and emphysema at the same time. You can start with chronic bronchitis and then develop emphysema or symptoms of both can appear at about the same time. The tendency toward COPD seems to run in families. But whether a person has inherited a genetic tendency for COPD, or has developed it as a result of environmental and social issues, is a difficult call to make. For example, we know that children who grow up in a house where parents smoke have a history of childhood respiratory problems, and many patients who develop a COPD report frequent colds as children. Genetics may also play a part, however.

We also know that if there is a smoker in the family, the children tend to smoke. We're not certain then if this association of COPD is physiological, genetic, or just picked up culturally. It is not uncommon for several family members to have a range of pulmonary problems.

For example, my patient Mrs. Carter has severe emphysema and requires oxygen for more than eighteen hours each day. Her daughter Denise had asthma as a child and because she saw how cigarettes affected her mother, never started the hard-to-break habit. When Denise gets a cold, it tends to develop into a heavy cough and she calls me for antibiotics. Happily, her pulmonary function tests are well within the normal range. Her Uncle James, who has smoked since his teens, is also one of my patients. I am following him for chronic obstructive bronchitis, and early signs of emphysema. While Denise, her mother, and Uncle James have different forms of COPD, I suspect that there is probably an underlying pulmonary weakness that is shared by the family, but the most serious problems appear to be limited to those who smoke cigarettes.

COPD is a progressive disease and we have mapped the progression in a series of four stages. Each has its own set of symptoms, laboratory test results, and treatment protocols.

Stage 0—At Risk

Usually characterized by chronic cough and phlegm production and/or shortness of breath, pulmonary function is still normal. Most people are completely unaware that trouble is brewing, but this is exactly the time to begin periodic medical care. Patients often feel that they are wasting a doctor's time for "annoying" symptoms like a chronic cough. On the contrary, we are delighted to see people before less treatable problems develop.

Stage I—Mild COPD

In addition to cough and mucus production, we now see mild airflow impairment. At this stage, many patients are still unaware that they have problems, while others notice that they are coughing more. Although they may become breathless more easily, they frequently attribute the feeling to normal aging. They are wrong.

Stage II—Moderate COPD

Shortness of breath forces patients to seek medical attention. Cough may or may not be a problem, but pulmonary function decreases sharply from normal. In addition to chronic shortness of breath, there are episodes of acute exacerbation and even a simple cold can cause a marked worsening of symptoms that may require hospitalization.

Stage III—Severe COPD

Symptoms are constant and severe. Breathing is difficult, even when sitting quietly. Daily activities are difficult and pulmonary function is seriously compromised. It can be hard to walk across the room, wash dishes, or even drive a car. Exacerbations can be frequent and life-threatening. At this point, I expect to see signs of right heart failure known as Cor Pulmonale. Two major developments contribute to this strain on the right heart. First, the destruction of lung tissue reduces the number of blood vessels through which the right heart can pump blood through the lungs; secondly, the oxygen carried by the blood is reduced due to the severe lung disease and this hypoxia causes a reflex constriction of the pulmonary vessels. This reflex constriction responds well to oxygen therapy, which is usually recommended at this stage.

When patients come to me and I have to tell them they have emphysema, they often have already lost a great deal of their lung function. But emphysema is a disease that grows silently for many years, and if we can catch it earlier, with early diagnosis and treatment, we can prevent or forestall further damage.

Certainly, the most important factor in dealing with COPD of any kind is smoking cessation. If you are smoking and are short of breath, it would be wonderful for you to quit. It will be so much harder to keep you healthy and strong if you continue cigarette smoking. Not infrequently, people come to me so sick that they need immediate hospitalization and this forces them into a nonsmoking environment. After two weeks with oxygen therapy and IVs, they've frequently gone cold turkey on cigarettes. When they come out, they are actually in a very good position never to go back to smoking again. I hope, however, that it won't take a medical crisis to help you stop smoking. In Chapter 8, I'll take you through a supportive smoking cessation program that has a high success rate for my patients.

Asthma: A Disease on the Rise

A disease that affects more than 7 percent of Americans, asthma is an episodic inflammation of the airways with attacks that make breathing difficult. The number of Americans with asthma rose a staggering 84 percent between 1982 and 1994. Even more troubling, deaths from asthma more than doubled between 1977 and 1991. We'll look into possible causes later in this chapter.

Asthma in Women

Doctors have known for some time that women have higher rates of asthma than men. Additionally, recent research now indicates that the severity of asthma symptoms vary with the menstrual cycle. These studies have shown that 40 percent of women experience increased wheezing premenstrually and are 4X more likely to have to go to an ER for an asthma attack.

Changes in breathing and lung function are a normal part of menstruation. During the premenstrual period the work of breathing increases 30 percent, the result in changes routinely seen during pregnancy. The airways become more sensitive and are more prone to narrowing. To complicate matters further women with asthma have reduced response to their normally effective bronchodilators. Fortunately, inhaled corticosteroids are still effective during the menstrual cycle for relieving inflammation and keeping the airways from narrowing. For some women it can be very helpful to keep a calendar of symptoms. If wheezing and shortness of breath occur frequently during menstruation, your doctor can add or increase inhaled steroids in addition to bronchodilators at this vulnerable time.

Asthmatic attacks are not subtle events. Unlike COPD, where the symptoms creep up on you, the acute shortness of breath, wheezing, and coughing of asthma make their presence known very quickly and early. Most people develop asthma as children. Some find that it disappears by their teenage years, but at least 50 percent of adults with childhood asthma still experience asthma symptoms. Asthma that goes away during the teenage years may still be present at a subclinical level, and can be retriggered in adulthood by a bad cold or exposure to strong irritants or allergens.

For example, one of my patients had asthma as a child and still remembers the frightening nighttime trips to the emergency room. When she reached fifteen, the asthma seemed to go away, and stayed away for more than twenty years. One night there was a large explosion and fire in her apartment building, and although she wasn't burned or injured, she was exposed to heavy smoke. After this incident, her asthma returned full force and her two children, who had been healthy, both developed severe asthma.

The Unimaginable Event

On September 11, 2001, the collapse of the World Trade Center and the massive blaze at Ground Zero exposed tens of thousands of people to an unprecedented level of airborne pollutants. It was a catastrophic event unlike anything in our experience. From the first day, we have been gathering data on the health impact of New Yorkers.

In most fires, one of the primary concerns is the outgassing of compounds as they burn. In the WTC collapse, the air itself was black with particulate matter. The level of suspended particles was so high that the sky was as dark as night. People reported that the air was suffocating and that they found it difficult to even swallow.

Health problems have continued in the months that followed. The illness known as the "WTC Syndrome" is characterized by a chronic cough, sore throat, and gastrointestinal problems. Doctors suspect that the refluxlike

(continued)

symptoms can be traced to the swallowing of large irritating particles generated in the collapse.

The first concern of the medical teams dealing with the disaster was the more than 8,000 firefighters, policemen, and rescue workers who rushed to the scene. Currently, all the rescuers involved in the disaster are being followed carefully for health problems. In addition, doctors are studying small groups of people exposed to some of the greatest concentrations of pollutants to identify trends. For example, 100 firefighters were given pulmonary challenge tests and it was found that 25 percent had hyperreactivity of their airways, a finding usually associated with asthma. However, researchers are quick to point out that this type of irritable airways, which presents without a history or sign of previous asthma, does not necessarily mean an individual is now asthmatic. Doctors are now looking to see if the WTC rescue workers go on to develop occupational asthma or other types of environmental pulmonary disorders.

There has been a great deal of understandable concern about the toxic airborne substances (such as heavy metals and asbestos) that were released in the carnage on the people who live and work in downtown New York. Our first concern is for people with known pulmonary problems, such as asthma and bronchitis, and they are being carefully monitored. There are also ongoing studies on the pulmonary function of healthy people who were exposed (and continue to be exposed) to pollution from the WTC collapse.

An Epidemic of Asthma

We don't know why asthma rates have soared in recent years. It may be that we're being exposed to more pollutants, or that there may be new irritants in the environment or in the home that we're not aware of. Asthma seems to run in families, and most asthmatics have a close relative with the disorder. Many cases of asthma are linked to allergies, and there is a close relationship between a history of allergies and development of asthma.

Asthma: Close-Up and Personal

Asthma is a chronic inflammatory disorder of the airways, caused by our reaction to allergens and irritants in the environment. When the airways come in contact with these triggers, they respond with a series of cellular and biochemical changes that lead to the contraction of the smooth muscles that line the interior of the airways, a swelling of the bronchial tissue, and the production of thick mucus.

The result is difficulty in breathing, chest tightness, and coughing. These episodes usually can end spontaneously or with medication, but they can also be severe and life-threatening. In past years, we viewed asthma as a completely reversible disease— that is, we thought that once the acute symptoms ended, lung function and airway architecture returned to normal. More recently, we have come to recognize that over time asthma can cause permanent abnormalities in the health and function of the lungs.

These slow changes, which include permanent thickening of the airways, are known as remodeling. It is a process that changes asthma from an occasional problem into a constant issue for pulmonary health. We now see asthma patients whose lung pathology and symptoms are indistinguishable from COPD. It is this remodeling that we want to avoid with the preventive strategies offered in *Life and Breath*.

Asthma usually begins in younger patients and can last a

lifetime, but it can appear at any age. The symptoms of asthma are not always clearly apparent. For example, episodes of coughing that last for up to several hours and recur for weeks can actually be a first sign of asthma.

The Four Stages of Asthma

The issue of permanent pulmonary changes from asthma is so important that we classify stages of asthma according to frequency as well as severity of symptoms and lung function.

Stage 1—Mild Intermittent Asthma

Symptoms occur less than twice a week during the day, and last for several hours to several days. Nighttime symptoms occur less than twice a month. Between episodes there are no problems and lung function is normal.

Stage 2—Mild Persistent Asthma

Symptoms occur more than twice a week, but not more than once a day. In other words, you feel tightness and wheezing every day, but episodes are limited to one event each day. Symptoms can be severe enough that you have to stop whatever you are doing to get breathing under control. Nighttime symptoms occur more than twice a month and lung function declines slightly.

It's important to recognize that asthmatic attacks in mild persistent asthma can be severe and life-threatening. In fact, a study published in *Pediatric Pulmonology* found that 30 percent of asthma fatalities occurred in patients with mild asthma.

Stage 3—Moderate Persistent Asthma

Symptoms are part of daily life and develop more than once a week at night. Acute attacks occur more than twice a week and can last for days. Exacerbations are severe enough to interfere with daily activities, causing absence from school or work. Pulmonary function levels can decline fairly sharply, reflecting the impact of persistent bronchial constriction.

Stage 4—Severe Persistent Asthma

Symptoms of wheezing, chest tightness, and cough are constant during both day and night. It is difficult to participate in daily activities and quality of life is compromised. Work, school, social life, and even sleep become difficult. Acute attacks are frequent and pulmonary function is equal to that found in severe COPD. When people try to treat themselves unsuccessfully with over-the-counter products, they can find themselves fatally short of breath.

What Is Happening During an Asthmatic Attack

The airways of the asthmatic becomes inflamed from known irritants such as cleaning fluids or cold air. The smooth muscles of the asthmatic airways are hyperactive. It takes very little to set them off and when they become irritated, they become narrowed.

Specialized cells that are in the airways release substances called histamine, leukotrienes, and prostaglandins, all of which combine to create pulmonary havoc. They stimulate mucous glands to secrete thick mucus, which blocks up the airways. These mediators also cause blood vessels to become swollen and

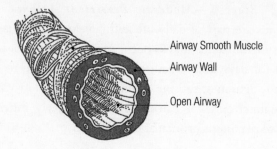

The healthy airway is open, allowing air to move easily in and
out of the lungs.

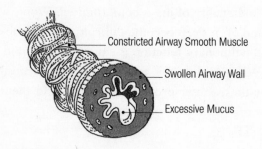

With asthma, airways are inflamed, swollen, and blocked with mucus.
In addition, contraction of the surrounding smooth muscle further
narrows the airway, increasing difficulty of breathing.

leaky and provoke the smooth airway muscles to constrict. The
net sum result of these changes is to narrow the airways so significantly that you simply cannot breathe in or out. Air gets trapped
in the lungs because smaller airways are obstructed or collapsed
and you can't exhale completely. As a result of lung overinflation,
the diaphragm is pulled down so you can't inhale efficiently.

During the '90s, we saw a frightening rise in asthma deaths,
and the American Lung Association launched a major public

education campaign to teach parents, children, and teachers how to prevent and manage attacks. After a decade of disturbing numbers, we are now seeing a real drop in asthma fatalities—a drop that we credit to better education and better treatment of asthma throughout the country.

Asthmatics are particularly sensitive to certain factors in the environment. For example, in the outdoors, simple cold air is a very well-known trigger for asthma. Pollen, pet dander, dust, ozone, and household cleaning solutions are also common triggers for hyperresponsive airways. While more women than men are diagnosed with asthma, it may be more severe in men. A study from the Bellevue Hospital Asthma Clinic found that asthmatic men had lower lung function, more visits to the emergency room, and showed less of a response to medication intended to open blocked airways. Asthma tends to become worse at night and appears to be caused by both environmental and physiological factors. Bedrooms have the highest concentration of dust mites, whose allergens are among the most frequent causes of asthma symptoms. These microscopic insects burrow into carpets and bedding, hide under the bed, and bury themselves in the folds of curtains. Eight hours of close exposure to concentrations of these microscopic creatures during the night can be a significant trigger for asthma.

Physical changes associated with natural biological rhythms may play an equally important role. Researchers have shown that sleep increases airway sensitivity, leading to bronchoconstriction. The body continually releases an anti-inflammatory substance, cortisol. There is, however, a natural nighttime fall in cortisol levels, which in asthmatics may lead to increased airway inflammation. With environmental controls and preventive medication, nighttime asthma can become manageable. Chapter Nine will explain exactly how to accomplish these strategies.

Developing Asthma as an Adult

Adult asthma can appear with a change of health status, such as after surgery, following a bad flu, or even during pregnancy. Jacqueline came from a family with allergies, but never had a problem with either allergies or asthma. At the start of her second pregnancy, she developed a chronic cough. During pregnancy, there are two people to be considered. If there is a drop in the mother's oxygen level, then the baby's oxygen can be compromised. Although we never like to load up a pregnant woman with medication, it is essential to manage the asthma of pregnancy, which can be fatal to both mother and child. I treated Jacqueline with bronchodilators and anti-inflammatory inhalers and both she and her baby did beautifully. Jacqueline continued to have asthma symptoms for the next six to seven years, but they became increasingly mild and infrequent as time passed. By the time her son was eight, her asthma was a distant memory.

Not infrequently, adult asthma is exacerbated or triggered by factors in the workplace. Although Jolene was barely thirty, she suffered from both asthma and bronchitis. She came to me because she was convinced that her job was the cause of all her problems. Jolene was an exotic dancer, and performed with a 30-lb. boa constrictor named Buddy around her neck. She only developed symptoms on the days she worked at the local topless club. She wondered if it was the weight of the snake on her

shoulders or an allergy to his scales that was causing her asthmatic symptoms. At this point, I moved onto the only area I
felt was certain ground. "Most animal allergies are associated
with warm-blooded mammals and Buddy is neither," I told her
with all the authority I could muster. Looking at the video that
Jolene provided, I saw the more likely cause of her problem.
Although she wore a costume so skimpy it would give anyone
bronchitis in cold weather, I could also see the club was dense
with cigarette smoke. Since Jolene and I agreed that a smoke-
free topless club was not a realistic option, she decided to
change careers, but Buddy remained as the family pet.

Asthmatics are not more susceptible to colds, but when they
do develop them, their colds can be more severe. A study from
The Queen's Medical Centre in Nottingham, England, found
that asthmatics tended to develop a lingering cough and shortness of breath from routine colds. To prevent these coughs
from developing into full-blown bronchitis, many pulmonologists prescribe antibiotics for patients who have caught even
simple colds. Although antibiotics are not effective against cold
viruses, the coughing may be due to secondary bacterial infection of cold-produced mucus. Colds and flus can cause permanent decline in lung status, and using antibiotics may prevent
this type of irreversible destruction.

Can Asthma Become a Form of COPD?

There has been a great deal of debate about whether or not
asthma should be included under the COPD umbrella. Both
chronic bronchitis and emphysema have been considered irreversible. The symptoms can be controlled, but the underly-

ing disease process is always there, silently decreasing lung function.

Historically, asthma has been regarded as completely reversible. Once the bronchoconstriction relaxed, we believed that lung function returned to normal levels. But large population studies reported changes in the lungs of adult asthmatics that were indistinguishable from those shown in patients with COPD. We saw that over time, undertreated or uncontrolled asthma caused irreversible lung damage and that, in fact, the symptoms would never fully leave. While doctors continue to argue about the merits of lumping and splitting these diagnoses, there is no doubt that many asthmatics can go on to develop the same pathologic changes as patients with other forms of chronic obstructive pulmonary disease. What this means to me as a physician and to you as a patient is that we need to work together to keep asthma inflammation under the best possible control, in order to avoid developing irreversible damage.

Asthma and Smoking

Asthmatics often have an aversion to smoke, but many others are smokers themselves. Interestingly, they often find it intolerable to be in a room with other smokers, and often they will go into a nonsmoking environment to smoke comfortably. Studies in England found that 50 percent of asthmatics in the U.K. continue to smoke cigarettes. It is never good to smoke, but asthma and smoking is a terrible combination, one that many patients just don't want to admit. At their peril, unfortunately.

In recent years, we have learned that asthma attacks are often preceded by very silent signs that we can detect with a simple device called a peak flow meter. This is a handheld instrument that can be used in your home to measure peak flow rates (the maximum speed at which air can be blown out of your lung). If the peak flow meter numbers start to trend downward, it is a sign that the airways are beginning to get into trouble. This can be a signal for you to increase your medication and call your doctor.

It's Not All in Your Head

There is a long tradition of considering psychological factors when dealing with asthma. Most doctors agree that stress, depression, or anxiety can trigger or worsen an asthma attack. But I tend to cringe at the idea that emotional problems can cause asthma. To me, that is blaming the victim for biochemical changes that are beyond their control. Personal issues, such as job pressures or a divorce, can make asthma worse, and asthma itself can produce a great deal of anxiety. It is essential that you understand that asthma is the result of hypersensitive airways, not emotional problems. For example, I have been caring for Hillary Bernstein, an accountant, for more than five years. She had been doing very well, when in late March, she developed persistent nighttime asthma attacks that sent her to the emergency room three times in as many weeks. When she came into my office, I could see the anxiety in her face. I tried to isolate what factors could be causing her symptoms. Frequently, a new home, a new pet, or construction in the workplace can produce asthma triggers. But none of these were relevant for Hillary. Then I asked her if there were any changes or problems in her family. She admitted that her mother had become increasingly frail in the past few weeks and this was the busy season for accountants. As she spoke about these issues, her coughing increased. I treated her with a fast-acting inhaler, then took her into an empty examining room to lie down and give her a chance to relax. I turned out the lights and pulled the curtain around to give her privacy. I assured her that I was right next door, and would check on her every ten minutes. When I came back, Hillary was asleep. An hour later when she woke up, her breathing had eased. The family and job pressures had triggered the attack, and the opportunity to relieve stress had allowed the medication to work.

If you already have asthma, emotional pressures can promote an attack as well as increase the frequency and severity of the symptoms. Because they can also depress the respiratory system, most pulmonologists do not prescribe tranquilizers for anxiety-related asthma problems. In Chapter Nine, I'm going to look at relaxation strategies such as yoga and biofeedback that can break the asthma/stress cycle.

Asthma as a Family Affair

Asthma, which can appear at any time during childhood, often announces itself during or after a bad respiratory infection. Usually, an asthmatic child has a history of allergies, and there is asthma and allergy in the family. Because it can be difficult, but not impossible, to do pulmonary function tests in children under the age of five, the diagnosis is frequently made on the basis of symptoms such as cough and shortness of breath, as well as with the help of the medical history of both the child and the parents. In infants, asthmalike symptoms can also be due to the problems induced by congenital heart disease, cystic fibrosis, and gastric reflux. These diagnoses need to be eliminated before the diagnosis of asthma can be established.

Younger children tend to have more severe asthma attacks, probably because their airways are smaller and have a tendency to collapse.

In children over the age of five, doctors can usually confirm the diagnosis of asthma with pulmonary function tests. Allergies are almost always associated with childhood asthma. Dust mites, pet dander, and cockroach antigens are the most frequent culprits. I also want to point out that children who grow up in a household where adults smoke are three times more likely to develop asthma. Following guidelines for healthy indoor air quality in Chapter 10 should significantly relieve breathing problems.

Chapter 4

The Causes of COPD

There is no debate. Over 40,000 studies have shown that cigarette smoking is a major cause of pulmonary death and disease. It is estimated that one in five deaths in the United States is due to tobacco-related illnesses. More than 440,000 people die each year from diseases directly related to smoking, and it is considered the single most preventable cause of premature death in the United States. It has been estimated that a heavy smoker at age twenty-five will have a 25 percent shorter lifespan than a nonsmoker of the same age. Other studies show that smokers have twice the overall mortality rate of nonsmokers. There are other factors that contribute to COPD, but chronic obstructive lung disease as we know it today would probably not exist without the epidemic of smoking in our time.

The costs to society are equally troubling. Direct medical costs for cigarette-related illness are more than $50 billion a year. If you add the cost of lost work and productivity, the price tag rises to $97 billion.

It is encouraging that the prevalence of cigarette smoking has declined slowly and steadily since the first Surgeon General's report on smoking and health was published in 1964. In 1965, 52 percent of men and 34 percent of women over the age of eighteen were smokers. By 1991, just 28 percent of men and 24 percent of women were still smoking cigarettes. Even the average number of cigarettes smoked a year dropped from 4,300 in 1963 to 2,600 in 1992. These encouraging numbers are offset by the number of new teenage smokers each year. Every day 3,000 additional teenagers start smoking. In addition, about 20 percent of high school seniors are smokers.

Cigarette smoke is composed of gases, vapors, and particles. This is due to the combustion of both the tobacco and the paper that surrounds the cigarette. As with any fire, the burning of organic material produces gases as well as liquids and solid particles composed of a large array of different chemicals. Many compounds like formaldehyde are irritating, while others like cyanide are poisons. Some of these chemicals have very specific effects, while others are just inflammatory. Some will cause smooth muscle to contract, while others like carbon monoxide don't damage the lungs directly, but combine with hemoglobin in the blood so oxygen cannot be carried. This makes the job of the lung, which is to deliver oxygen to the body, all the harder.

In addition to the production of more than 4,000 unhealthy chemicals, cigarette smoke provokes the release of millions of free radicals. These unstable molecules are routinely produced by the body as by-products of normal metabolism, a kind of cellular trash. Free radicals are constantly being produced, when we digest food, walk in the sun, or fight off infections.

Free radicals are molecules with a missing electron; they are unhappy molecules. They crash into and around the cells, looking for an extra electron to provide the stability they crave. In the process, they damage fragile cell walls, preventing waste products from getting out and blocking nutrients and oxygen from getting in.

Once inside the cell, free radicals disrupt DNA formation and provoke the production of irritating and inflammatory enzymes and hormones. Thankfully, there is a natural defense mechanism to free radicals in our body, a unique defense system that deploys antioxidants to stop or limit free radical development and activity. The body produces compounds such as catalase or superoxide dismutase (SOD) that stop destruction caused by free radicals. These agents give the out of control molecules the electrons they want so badly. Once the free radicals are neutralized, they cease to be a problem. For additional antioxidant help, the body also enlists antioxidants in the diet, such as vitamins A, C, and E.

Under ideal conditions, the number of free radicals in the body is kept under control by the antioxidants in the food or those manufactured internally. But environmental factors, such as smoking, pollution, or the physiological events of asthmatic or bronchitic attacks, provoke the development of millions of free radicals in levels higher than the body can ever handle.

Every puff of cigarette smoke sends literally trillions of free radicals down into the lungs. The buildup of these free radicals creates a situation known as *oxidative stress* that provokes the body into producing wave after wave of inflammatory compounds. This phenomenon provokes the release of additional compounds, including leukotrienes and prostaglandins, which promote bronchial constriction as well as mucus production.

To protect vital cell functions, cells have the capacity to turn on defensive mechanisms releasing another set of compounds called transcription factors. One of these is known as AP1, which has the ability to dissolve collagen and elastin fibers. In healthy situations, these scavenger enzymes keep the body free of debris and damaged tissue, but when overproduced will destroy healthy elastin that is, as we've seen, essential for strong and flexible lungs.

Epidemiological studies have shown that people whose diets were high in well-known antioxidants such as vitamin C and E have a reduced risk and rate of COPD and asthma, and we're going to talk a great deal about that in Chapter Six, "Eat Right, Breathe Easy."

The Dynamics of the Smoker's Cough

Chronic bronchitis, which is one of the most common forms of COPD, is felt to be the end result of episodes of inflammation of the airways from cigarette smoking or pollution. When the lung is repeatedly exposed to cigarette smoke, a number of changes result, all bad. In the larger airways, the mucous glands become larger, more active, and start to appear in places they normally don't go. This creates an increase in mucus production that is associated with a constant and chronic cough. In addition, the tall columnar cells of the airway surface lose their important cilia, those fine hairlike structures that propel mucus, bacteria, and pollutants out of the airways. This leads to accumulation of foreign material, which produces inflammation and infection.

This now signals the immune system to send in white blood cells that release enzymes to destroy the invaders. In the process, the large airways undergo changes known as remodeling. The effect of continual white blood cell battles causes the airways to become thickened, scarred, and irritable, a combination that leads to decreased airway diameter. As a result of this remodeling, it is harder to breathe easily and the lungs become increasingly sensitive to irritants. In the smaller airways farther down the bronchial tree, similar problems occur, leading to increased airway resistance.

When we wash out the lungs of cigarette smokers, there can be 100 times as many white blood cells there to protect the lungs as there are in healthy nonsmokers. In the right numbers, neutrophils play an important role in preventing infection. When they are there in too great a number, they provoke the release of compounds that cause destruction and inflammation.

Emphysema—and Smoking

Emphysema in general is a more serious disease of the lungs. As we've learned, emphysema affects the alveoli, the tiny air sacs at the end of the bronchial tree. The inflammation and destruction in these air sacs results in crippling breathing problems. One of the major supporting structures of the alveoli is elastin. This is the fiber that keeps lung tissue taut and prevents the lungs from overexpanding. When there is inflammation from cigarette smoke or infection from bacteria, the body sends white blood cells to engulf and destroy the foreign material. In the process, these white blood cells release enzymes such as elastase that can break down elastin and collagen fibers. As a result, the scaffolding of the lungs is destroyed.

Normally, these enzymes serve a useful purpose, clearing the body of dead bacteria and old damaged connective fibers. But when there is constant inflammation from cigarette smoke, there is an overproduction of elastin-destroying enzymes. Cigarette smoke provokes the body to build up white blood cells, which also contain elastase, and it is one of those enzymes that destroys unhealthy tissue.

It would be strange to think that the body constantly produces a substance that can destroy its own tissues without a control system to limit the damage. And in fact there is a control, another body chemical called alpha-1 antitrypsin. The destruction of elastin by elastase is controlled by the presence of this other inhibitor that stops elastase from destroying healthy connective tissue fibers. Research has shown that cigarette smoke inhibits or damages the development and activity of alpha-1 antitrypsin. Consequently, elastase activity is unchecked and healthy elastin is destroyed. Not only does cigarette smoke create oxidative stress that damages the lung, it actually provokes the body to destroy healthy connective tissue while destroying its natural protection.

The Damage Continues

Among the 4,000 poisons and toxins in cigarette smoke, nicotine, the main addictive component, is actually a constrictor of smooth muscle. This means, in addition to hooking the body on smoking, nicotine causes the airways to constrict and limit the amount of air an individual can either inhale or exhale.

Smoking does not directly cause asthma, but the tobacco contains many irritants like nicotine that stimulate the smooth muscle that surrounds our airways. As a result, cigarette smoke will provoke asthmatic attacks in sensitive lungs.

There is a common misconception that pipes and cigars are

less damaging than cigarettes, and they have been promoted as a way of weaning people away from cigarettes. Pipe and cigar smoke contains all the same tar and gases that are in cigarettes. If you inhale deeply enough and smoke enough of them, you will get the same quantities of irritants that you do in cigarettes—and have the same medical problems as with cigarettes. In addition, keep in mind there is also a greater frequency of upper respiratory cancers in pipe and cigar smokers. The irritating by-products of smoke stay longer and tend to accumulate in the mouth, tongue, and lips of people who use these alternative forms of tobacco.

With so many toxic effects, there is no surprise that there is a relationship between the amount of smoke inhaled over a lifetime and the health consequences of cigarette smoking; we call this a dose response. We measure smoking levels in terms of the number of packs per day smoked and the number of years smoked. It probably comes as no surprise to learn that the more you smoke, the more health problems you are likely to develop.

When we are trying to find out whether a person is at risk for cigarette-related diseases, even before we've examined them or done a chest X ray, we quantify the amount of cigarettes they have been exposed to. We do this by evaluating the number of pack years, that is the number of years a person has smoked times the average number of packs they smoked per day.

Most cigarette smokers will smoke on average a pack a day. That's the average fix a smoker needs to keep his habit satisfied. If you started smoking at fifteen and are now forty, this means you've smoked for twenty-five years. If you smoked an average of one pack of cigarettes a day, then you have twenty-five pack years exposure.

I always like to compare smoking history to savings accounts. The earlier you start saving, the more money you wind up with when you retire. Unfortunately, with cigarette smoking, this has a negative value. The earlier you start smoking, the more damage and the more pack years you've had when you become an adult. People who start smoking when they are ten years old can have a frightening number of pack years by the time they reach forty. To cite a ballpark figure, twenty pack years is usually the amount of smoking exposure at which we start to see real health consequences develop.

Who Gets COPD?

Not everyone who smokes develops emphysema or chronic bronchitis. There is a feeling that the resistance or susceptibility to emphysema is to some degree inherited. Although we realize there is a hereditary factor to almost all of COPD, it has been well characterized in only a small number of individuals who develop hereditary emphysema caused by the so-called alpha-1 antitrypsin deficiency.

This type of emphysema was discovered in Sweden in 1963 by two physicians, Sten Eriksson and Carl-Bertil Laurell. One was a clinician and the other ran a clinical laboratory. They noticed that out of thousands of tests they analyzed, they found the same little bump known as alpha-1 was missing in several individuals. The clinician, Eriksson, went to the hospital where these patients had been admitted, got their charts, and reviewed them. What he found was that the health problems that characterized all these patients were that they had chronic lung disease. The proteins that made up the little bump were analyzed and it was concluded that the major component was alpha-1 antitrypsin. In other words, the chemical analysis of their blood showed they were lacking this very important substance.

As noted earlier, alpha-1 antitrypsin is an enzyme-antagonist that blocks the activity of enzymes such as elastase. It prevents the enzyme which digests elastin from autodigesting the elastin that is the major component of the scaffolding of the lung.

Why Is This Important?

Emphysema is usually a disease of middle age and starts around age fifty. If you look at patients over fifty with emphysema, only about one out of a hundred have this alpha-1 antitrypsin deficiency. However, if you look at patients under fifty who develop emphysema, nearly half of them have the alpha-1 antitrypsin deficiency. In other words, the lack of this anti-enzyme predisposes you to premature emphysema.

Scientists have identified several defective genes that either singly or in combination are responsible for abnormal forms of alpha-1 antitrypsin. If one such gene is present, the alpha-1 antitrypsin levels are lower or the enzyme performs poorly. If both genes are defective, then the alpha-1 antitrypsin is nearly entirely absent. Interestingly, the free radicals that are produced by cigarette smoke inactivate the alpha-1 antitrypsin enzyme. If you have a deficiency of the gene, and you smoke, your levels of antitrypsin are simply not sufficient to protect you against autodestruction.

The Healthy Cigarette?

Just as the alchemists' goal was to turn lead into gold, the tobacco industry has been trying to produce a healthy cigarette. We don't know if they are sincere in their efforts to market healthier products, but it is clear that they want to continue to sell cigarettes.

The solid particles in cigarette smoke known as tar are the source of many toxins and carcinogens. In the low-tar cigarette, you remove some carcinogenic tar as well as a certain amount of nicotine. In order to get the same "hit" from a cigarette, we have found the people inhale more deeply and smoke more cigarettes to get the nicotine their body craves. The end result? They wind up with the same amount of tar and nicotine and may even spend more for low-tar cigarettes.

Secondhand Smoke

Each time a person lights up a cigarette, deadly toxic chemicals, such as formaldehyde, benzene, and carbon monoxide, are released into the air. These toxins not only affect the smoker, they can harm nonsmokers who are in the same environment. Known as secondhand smoke, it can cause increased mortality from lung cancer and heart disease in nonsmokers.

There are actually two forms of secondhand smoke. Sidestream smoke comes from the tip of the burning cigarette and flows right into the air. Mainstream smoke is exhaled from the smoker. Sidestream smoke is actually higher in harmful ingredients than smoke that has been filtered by someone else's lungs. Inhaled smoke first passes through the cigarette, its filters, and deposits more chemicals into the lungs before it is exhaled. Sidestream smoke contains all the products of the un-filtered combustion.

Secondhand smoke is particularly harmful for children. Cig-arette smoking during pregnancy has been associated with the development of asthma in the child. Researchers from the University of Southern California, following 6,000 children, found that more than 30 percent of those youngsters whose mothers smoked during pregnancy had episodes of wheezing. In addition, growing up in a smoke-filled home has been linked to high rates of bronchitis, asthma, and impaired lung function as adults. Researchers have reported that healthy chil-dren had twice the incidence of acute respiratory infections if their parents smoked. For example, it is estimated that up to 300,000 cases of bronchitis and pneumonia in children under eighteen months old are associated with cigarettes in their home.

The American Lung Association has led antismoking efforts with great success. Both state and local laws now limit smoking in restaurants, hospitals, schools, and offices in most states. Smoking is now banned on all foreign and domestic flights, buses, and trains originating in the United States. Eliminating the number of places where smoking is permitted is a win-win situation. In addition to protecting the health of nonsmokers, it will make it harder for smokers to continue their habit and may be just the nudge they need to quit.

Asthma: When You Suddenly Can't Breathe

Asthma frequently starts in childhood. Ninety percent of child-hood asthma is associated with allergies. Doctors believe that there is an inherited tendency to produce higher levels of an antibody known as Immunoglobulin E (IgE), which is directed against common allergens such as those associated with pets, dust, milk, and molds. About 50 percent of the time people find childhood asthma symptoms begin to disappear as they become teenagers. The reason for this is not clear. Some researchers suggest that as the airway grows the obstruction associated with childhood asthma becomes less important.

Adult onset asthma can begin at any age. Sometimes it is a return of childhood symptoms, while other adults develop asthma problems for the first time. Adult asthma can start following a viral infection, environmental exposure (such as a fire), workplace exposure, or can be due to definable allergies.

The allergy-related asthma attack usually has two phases. The first phase begins immediately after exposure to an allergen. The IgE antibody sites on mast cells (allergy cells chockfull of mediators) in the airways couple with the allergens. This activates the mast cells to release substances called mediators, including histamine, a cell mediator that causes the airways to constrict, provoking both mucus production and swelling in the lining of the airways. This first stage lasts minutes to a few hours and causes symptoms of wheezing and chest tightness. The second phase begins several hours after the first phase ends. Mast cells also release compounds such as leukotrienes, mediators that are the metabolic by-products of arachidonic acid, which are themselves breakdown products of cell walls damaged by inflammation. This cascade of events is associated with high levels of free radicals, and their effects are often delayed. Leukotrienes attract white blood cells to the airways that produce greater and longer-lasting problems of swelling, mucus production, and bronchoconstriction.

At this point, the airways, swollen, narrowed, and filled with mucus, find it increasingly difficult to allow air to move in and out of the lungs. This situation produces symptoms of wheezing, coughing, and shortness of breath that can last days and even weeks.

Asthmatic attacks can also be triggered by exposure to irritants such as formaldehyde, cigarette smoke, or even cold air. While IgE antibodies probably are not significant in the development of symptoms related to these triggers, the same mediators that form or are released as part of the allergic response play a prominent role in this "irritant" response. In irritant asthma, the nonallergic form of asthma, there is a release of mediators including leukotrienes and prostaglandins that produce precisely the same symptoms as allergic asthma.

The Role of Free Radicals in Asthma

Free radicals are by-products of normal metabolism—a kind of cellular trash. The inflammation produced in an asthmatic response generates the production of a large number of free radicals in the airways as a result of damage caused by the action of mediators. We've seen the destructive impact of these hyperactive molecules, creating havoc, breaking DNA strands, and altering normal enzymatic activities. The impact of these changes causes more inflammation and leads to increased bronchoconstriction and mucus production, resulting in higher levels of oxidative stress.

Epidemiological studies have shown that people who eat a diet high in fruits, vegetables, and fish have lower asthma rates than those that don't. Researchers believe that the antioxidant vitamins and bioflavinoids (naturally occurring agents that protect plants against insects and molds) in these foods block the development of free radicals, thus reducing oxidative stress levels. In Chapter Six, I will focus on the role of diet in pulmonary health and explain how to translate these scientific findings into pulmonary protective meals.

Whether provoked by irritants, allergens, or complicated by free radicals, over time we have seen a permanent change in the architecture of asthmatic airways. Known as remodeling, these irreversible changes can be indistinguishable from the damage we see in COPD. It is exactly this type of damage that we want to prevent.

Is Breathing Hazardous to Your Health?

In 1948, an air pollution crisis affected 40 percent of the residents of Donora, Pennsylvania. This small town was home to a zinc production plant, a sulfuric acid factory, and a full-service steel mill. On a cloudy, windless day, a fog rolled into the area. By the next day, the combination of still air, natural fog, and a witches' brew of emissions from the industrial smokestacks produced a dense black cloud hovering over the town. The air was dark and dense and it was impossible to see across the small streets. People began to cough and complain of sore throats and burning eyes. By the time the fog lifted, twenty people had died as a direct result of this air pollution crisis. A few years later, a deadly combination of warm still air and sulfur dioxide pollution resulted in 4,000 unanticipated deaths in London's famous "Killer Fog."

We have been concerned about the health impact of industrial pollution since the start of the industrial revolution. The overwhelming source of outdoor pollution today comes from the burning of fossil fuels such as natural gas, oil, and coal. Air pollution creates health problems by destroying lung tissue and weakening our defenses against disease. As you remember from Chapter Two, there is a sticky coating of mucus that lines our airways. It functions like flypaper to capture bacteria, dirt, and contaminants before they can enter the deep airways of the lungs. The epithelial columnar cells, equipped with tiny "hairs" called cilia, propel the mucus (and its trapped material) out of the body. Unfortunately, air pollution can paralyze or even destroy the cilia. As a result, "junk" builds up in the mucus that can overwhelm our immune system. To make matters worse, we try to defend ourselves from pollution by breathing less. Our airways narrow as a natural reflex to limit our intake of irritating compounds, making it more difficult to breathe.

The Fatal Four

While there are over 200 known pollutants, four specific compounds either singly or in combination, are of great concern for pulmonary health:

Nitrogen Dioxide (NO_2): This is a light brown gas that is formed when fossil fuels are burned at very high temperatures, such as those that are found in motor vehicles and power plants. You will find that the highest levels of NO_2 are at road level and when there is heavy traffic. A strong oxidant, NO_2 increases free radical levels in the body and can aggravate and provoke symptoms of allergy and asthma.

Some studies link high NO_2 levels to an increased risk of bronchitis and upper respiratory infections such as influenza in the community. The impact of NO_2 appears primarily on people with existing pulmonary problems, and not in healthy lungs. It can't be blamed for causing asthma and COPD, but it can certainly make symptoms worse.

The U.S. Environmental Protection Agency (EPA) set National Ambient Air Quality Standards (NAAQS) for NO_2 to an annual average of .053 parts per million. Fortunately, there are no localities in the United States that currently exceed this standard.

Outdoor Pollution in Your Home

In your kitchen, gas stoves also give off NO_2. If you have a gas stove, make sure there is a window open nearby when you cook. If you are replacing your current stove, look into an electric model. It can make a big impact in your indoor air quality.

Ozone (O_3): An especially nasty pollutant, ozone is also produced when NO_2 mixes with sunlight. This photochemical pollutant is a major source of free radicals in our environment, and ozone is the primary component of smog. Ozone levels have been rising steadily over the past forty years, a consequence of the increasing numbers of cars in the United States. Ozone levels rise in the morning and peak by midafternoon. At night when the sun goes down and traffic slows, the ozone levels decrease.

Studies have reported inflammation of the airway lining, wheezing, and an increase in hospital admissions for respiratory problems due to high ozone levels. The greatest degree of ozone exposure occurs in adults and children who are exercising outdoors. It has been shown that unhealthy levels of ozone can even impair the performance times of elite athletes. Long-term repeated exposure to high levels of ozone may lead to large reductions in lung function, inflammation of the lung lining, and increased respiratory distress.

Ozone levels are highest in warm weather. A study of long-term residents in Los Angeles (which has the highest ozone levels in the United States) found Angelenos as a group had a higher than expected decline in lung function.

Despite an improvement following the adoption of EPA standards, it has been difficult to keep pace with the increasing number of cars in our society. The most recent standards from the EPA strengthened acceptable ozone limits from .12 parts/million to .08 parts per million over an eight-hour period. The implementation of the new standards has been challenged in the courts. Researchers calculate that 270 counties in thirty-three states violate this new standard. It has been calculated that 117 million people living in these areas are at risk from the health effects of elevated ozone levels.

There are three particular groups of people who are affected by ozone:

- *People with Diagnosed Pulmonary Problems*—If you already have reduced lung function, the exposure to even "acceptable" levels of ozone may cause wheezing and chest tightness.
- *Healthy Responders*—These are otherwise healthy people who, for reasons not entirely clear, are sensitive to the irritative effects of ozone. Their airways constrict to relatively low levels of this pollutant. It is estimated that between 5 to

20 percent of healthy people have an increased sensitivity to ozone. There is currently no way to identify these people, but we do know that cigarette smoking will have an additive effect on airway damage.

■ *People Who Exercise Outdoors*—When we participate in sports, our breathing rate increases and as a result we breathe in more ozone than if we were just sitting or strolling in the sun.

Reducing Ozone Levels

Controlling individual exposure to ozone is not a do-it-yourself project. To reduce ozone air pollution, we need:

■ Stronger pollution controls for new cars

■ Cleaner fuel standards

■ Stricter pollution requirements for power plants, especially those built before 1977

Sulfur Dioxide (SO_2): This pollutant is formed when coal and oil are burned at high temperatures. Not unexpectedly, the highest levels of SO_2 are found in the areas where there are sizable electric utility companies that use large amounts of fossil fuels to produce power. SO_2 exposure has been linked to upper respiratory problems, a decrease in respiratory immunity, and aggravation of existing heart disease.

Epidemiological evidence has shown that SO_2 can cause problems in irritable airways. High levels of SO_2 have been linked to an increased incidence of colds and flus, especially in children and can aggravate cardiovascular disease. The current EPA standards for SO_2 are .50 parts/million averaged over three hours, 0.14 ppm over twenty-four hours, and .03 ppm annual arithmetic mean. There are currently thirty-three localities in the United States that exceed these levels.

Nationwide, electrical utilities produce more than 60 percent of the SO_2 in our air. Utility plants produce different levels of SO_2, depending on the fuel mix they use and the degree to which they have complied with pollution control measures. The power plants built before 1970 were exempted from the Clean Air Act Amendment of 1977. It was thought that there older plants would soon be replaced by newer and cleaner facilities. It didn't work out that way. Currently, 65 percent of utility plants were built before 1977, and some still generate four to ten times the SO_2 rate allowable for new plants.

Eliminating this loophole would force these older plants to install air pollution control devices. Not surprisingly, power plant industry officials are actively fighting increased regulations, claiming they will make power far more expensive. When balancing these costs, it is important to take into consideration the increased health care costs that can result from unacceptably high levels of SO_2 pollution.

Particulate Matter: Also known as PM, particulate matter is an umbrella term for a varying mix of dust and acid aerosols in the air. The solid portion is a mix composed of dirt, soil, pollen, mold, ashes, and soot. The acid aerosols are formed from by-products of other pollutants, such as sulfur dioxide and nitrogen oxides. PM pollution comes from a wide range of industry smokestacks, wood fires, mining, farming, and construction.

Doctors are particularly concerned about the very fine particle matter (less than 2.5 microns in diameter) that can be inhaled deeply into the airways. Studies throughout the world have linked PM to a range of serious health problems. We know that PM can be irritating to people with asthma, chronic bronchitis, and emphysema, as well as heart disease. A recent study showed a 17 percent increase in mortality rates in areas with higher concentrations of particulate matter. Interestingly, another study published in the *Journal of the American Medical Association* estimated PM causes 30,000 premature deaths in the United States each year. In fact, the researchers noted that city residents where PM levels are high face a long-term risk of lung cancer similar to that of someone living with a smoker. These are troubling findings when you remember that the highest levels of pollutants produced in the World Trade Center collapse were particulate matter. In fact, ongoing studies suggest that it is the PM inhaled by rescue workers that is the cause of the WTC syndrome we discussed earlier.

Relative Particle Size

(A micron is one millionth of a meter)

- Pollen, mold, spores—30 microns
- Household Dust—10 microns
- Red Blood Cell—7.5 microns
- Cat allergen—5 microns

Particles less than 5 microns can easily penetrate to the smallest airways, while those of greater size remain in the larger airways.

The good news is that outdoor air pollution levels have declined over the past twenty years. The bad news is that even at these lower levels, people with sensitive airways can still develop symptoms. If you have asthma or COPD, avoid high traffic areas during rush hour. If there is an air pollution alert, try to stay indoors with your windows shut, turn on the air conditioner, and let your air filter run continuously. See Chapters 10 and 11 for more tips on managing your environment.

We know that, either singly or in combination, cigarette smoke, pollution, and allergies cause different types of obstructive lung disease. In upcoming chapters, I'm going to look at ways to reduce these risk factors as well as reverse existing pulmonary problems.

Chapter 5

The Complete Chest Workup

Since I'm a pulmonary specialist, people generally don't come to me for a routine checkup. If you come to see me as a patient at Mt. Sinai Hospital, you probably have some specific pulmonary problem in mind. If you are a current or former smoker, you may be afraid of lung cancer or emphysema. You may have made the appointment because of a specific symptom, such as breathlessness or coughing. That symptom will be the starting point of my attempt to diagnose you. This is called the chief complaint and it's a one- or two-sentence description of the symptom that's bothering you.

Typically, shortness of breath in a person over fifty can be described as a slowly progressive problem. My patients who are in their fifties or sixties may have ignored this symptom for months or even years. They view that shortness of breath as part of normal aging. They slow down, saying to themselves, "Oh, I'm getting on in years. I do less, but then, so does everybody else." They are pleasantly surprised to learn that breathlessness need not be part of normal aging—and that proper diagnosis and treatment can restore strength and endurance.

To get more information about their breathlessness, I ask very simple questions. For example, how far can you walk on a flat surface without having to stop? If you are under sixty-five and can walk only one or two blocks without stopping, I begin to gain insight into the limitations of your pulmonary system. I also want to learn how many flights of stairs you can climb. Many city dwellers don't have stairs to climb in their home, so I ask about subway stairs. I want to find out if you have to stop between flights, in order to be comfortable. I ask you to think back two or three years to see if there has been any change in your activity level. For example, I want to know if you have been participating in sports or hobbies, but have found that now these activities are too much of an effort. Your answer will give me better insight into your physical condition.

Sometimes patients tell me that shortness of breath comes on in rapid, frightening episodes. These attacks often occur at night or with exposure to cold air or strong odors, such as perfumes or cleaning fluids. Such symptoms can also be triggered by allergens, such as pollens or pet hair. When attacks tend to be acute, I think of asthma rather than bronchitis or emphysema.

Chest tightness is another way that people perceive shortness of breath. Patients describe the sensation as a rope or a sheet that's tightly bound around the chest, making it difficult to take a breath. By and large, chest tightness is due to some of the same conditions that produce shortness of breath.

Patients who have chronic lung disease can develop secondary infections and can develop fever. When that happens, the shortness of breath becomes much more severe. They begin coughing more intensively, bringing up more phlegm. These are called acute exacerbations of the underlying lung problem, and they possibly represent a worsening of the disease.

The second most common complaint in my office is the symptom of coughing. The cough can be paroxysmal; in other words, coming on acutely. Alternatively, it can be chronic, present every day—annoying but not disabling.

Acute episodes of coughing that come on with shortness of breath can be another symptom of asthma. Frequently, the asthmatic cough will be dry, accompanied by a tickle in the back of the throat or some discomfort in the chest that provokes coughing.

Chest pain is another important, though infrequent, symptom of lung disease. You may be surprised to discover that lung tissue has no pain fibers. You can have terrible destruction of your lungs and not feel pain. When pain is present, it is often a sign of an infection or inflammation called pleurisy.

The lungs are covered with a thin mucous membrane called the pleura. One leaf of the pleura is attached to the lung itself and another leaf is plastered onto the surface of the chest wall. In between these two very thin layers of cells is a thin liquid layer called the pleural fluid. As we breathe, the pleural fluid provides a lubrication that allows the lungs to glide smoothly inside the chest, preventing damage from the ribs and the projections of the chest wall. When the pleura becomes inflamed from viral or bacterial infections such as pneumonia or as the result of a blood clot, it produces a sharp characteristic pain. Usually localized to one side of the chest, it hurts patients when they take a deep breath, cough, or sneeze. If it's persistent, the pleuritic pain can be a sign of serious underlying lung problems.

Most chest pain is not associated specifically with lung disease. The heart, the esophagus, and the chest wall (which consists of muscles, bones, and joints) can develop painful problems of their own. In a heart attack, the pain is usually in the center of the chest. Severe and frightening, the pain can migrate along the chest to the left shoulder, and then down to the left arm.

When the pain is the result of trouble in the esophagus, there is frequently a burning sensation in the middle of the chest. The discomfort usually is associated with large, spicy, or fatty meals. When the patient lies down at night to go to sleep, the peptic acid rolls back into the esophagus and essentially causes a burning of the tissue.

The most common causes of pain in the chest have to do with nonspecific problems such as trauma to the bones, muscles, or joints of the chest. For example, there are joints between the breastbone and ribs that can be arthritic, and painful.

Don't Be Scared Silent

Patients readily describe phlegm, shortness of breath, chest pain, and coughing to me, but are often hesitant about another symptom: coughing up blood. I usually wait well into the examination to ask about the symptom which seems to be so frightening that patients may deny it occurs or minimize its appearance. I don't want to minimize what could be a potentially serious problem, but most of the time, coughing up blood does not mean tuberculosis or cancer. The most common cause for hemoptysis (technical term for coughing up blood) is bronchitis, an inflammation of the airway. People who cough continuously put pressure on the tiny blood vessels in the airway, squeezing them so hard that some burst and a little bit of blood appears. When you cough, the blood appears as streaks in the phlegm. On the other hand, coughing up blood, particularly in the context of a person who's a middle-aged smoker, can also be a sign of lung cancer or pneumonia. As a result, anyone who complains of it, even though the chances are that it is not indicative of a life threatening condition, should have a chest X ray and further examination.

Clues into the Present Lie in the Past

Once I get a clear idea of your current symptoms, I go into a more general evaluation of your history. Called the past medical history, it takes us away from the lungs and goes over all those other major diseases that could interact or cause symptoms similar to lung disease. Heart disease or gastrointestinal problems, such as gallbladder and acid reflux, can produce symptoms similar to but distinguishable from chronic lung disease.

We will also talk about previous surgeries and allergies and find out what medicine a patient is taking. Sometimes I ask a patient if they have lung disease and they'll say no. Then I'll ask them to list medications that they are taking and they'll name five drugs that are specific for asthma or chronic bronchitis. For example, Sophia came to me because she had episodes of coughing that were so intense that she burst a blood vessel in her eye. She denied having pulmonary problems, yet when I asked her about medication, she opened her purse to reveal no less than six products for asthma. Still, she denied having asthma. Her inhalers were "for allergies" and a well-known

bronchodilator was "to help me relax." Sophia had recently ar-
rived in the United States from Greece and the doctor who
had prescribed these medications was an equally new arrival
from Uzbekistan. I imagine that language barriers were just a
bit too much for both of them. When a patient is unaware if
they have chronic lung disease, though they're taking medication for it, they may not have been told of it, they may not
have asked about it, or they've chosen to ignore the fact that
they have these problems.

When I ask what medications you are taking, I also look for
any drugs that actually cause coughing. For example, beta
blocker medications such as Inderal, used for hypertension and
angina, will exacerbate symptoms that accompany asthma and
bronchitis. Angiotensin-converting enzyme (ACE) inhibitors
such as Captopril, which are also used for hypertension, can
cause coughs in and of themselves. I actually see quite a few patients whose chronic cough is solely the result of the use of
ACE inhibitors. Changing to another type of antihypertensive
medication may eliminate coughing spasms.

At this point in the examination, I feel I have built up
enough of a rapport with you to go into what pulmonologists
call "the forbidden zone"—smoking history. This is one of the
most important areas that we have to explore, because the presence or absence of a smoking history very definitely changes
the context in which we put the symptoms and the findings of
our examination.

I'll focus on the number of cigarettes, pipes, or cigars you
have used over the years. Most commonly, it will be cigarette
smoking. I ask, "Are you currently a smoker?" In other words,
are you still smoking? If you are not currently smoking but

have smoked in the past, I view you as an ex-smoker. Here the most important question is: "When did you stop?" It may be two minutes ago or five years ago and both answers give me additional helpful information.

Many of the complications of cigarette smoking diminish after you quit, while others are fixed. In other words, if you smoke up to a point and then quit completely, you will have a certain type of damage that remains with you for the rest of your life but progresses no further. Then there are problems, such as lung cancer, which may occur many years after the person has stopped smoking. Fortunately, there are benefits that start almost as soon as you stop smoking.

In addition to establishing when you stopped smoking, I will ask when you started. For most, it is between the ages of fifteen and twenty. It never fails to frighten me that a good number of people start before the age of fourteen. Interestingly, some people even consider themselves ex-smokers by the time they reach fifteen or sixteen. People usually don't start smoking after they've gone through their teenage years.

Whatever the smoking history, I can quantify the amount of damage you've potentially done by calculating the amount you have smoked. In order to do this, I will ask you to estimate the average number of cigarettes you smoked per day over the span of your lifetime. Obviously, that number varies from day to day and year to year. When you start smoking, you smoke a few cigarettes a day. When you try to quit, you cut down. But over the years there is an average and for most people that figure is somewhere between a half a pack to a pack a day. There are, of course, outliers, people who smoke a few cigarettes a week and those people who smoke four to five packs of cigarettes a day.

In order to figure out the total you have smoked, I calculate the number of years you have smoked (which is your current age, or the age at which you stopped, minus the age at which you started), and then multiply that by the average number of packs smoked per day. The number that is derived is called "pack years." For example, if you are forty years old and say, "I started when I was fifteen and am still smoking." I can calculate that you have smoked for twenty-five years. If you smoke on the average one pack a day, that means your lifetime burden of cigarettes is twenty-five pack years. If, on the other hand, you smoke two packs a day, your lifetime burden would be fifty pack years.

While no smoking level is without risk, most cigarette-related diseases (emphysema, heart disease, and lung cancer) usually manifest themselves in people after they've developed a burden of twenty pack years. Keep in mind the fact that this could be four packs a day for five years or one pack a day for twenty years.

The Life You've Lived

The next step in completing your history is to find out more about you . . . what you've done, where you've lived, what kind of jobs you've held, what you did in your free time are all factors that affect your lungs. For instance, 25 percent of the people who develop asthma as an adult can trace their pulmonary problems to their workplace environment, so I need to probe your working conditions.

When I begin my inquiries, people usually look at me somewhat curiously at first because there is a certain reluctance in people to discuss their jobs, hobbies, or housing. I try to clarify my questions by explaining that lifestyle issues that expose you to dust, fumes, chemicals, or any kind of product out of the ordinary can create long-term lung problems. For example, a patient named Fred Dummigan came to me with a bloody, pleural effusion. Talking with him, I learned that his hobby was taxidermy. An executive at a trucking company, taxidermy was his longtime hobby and passion. He hunted small animals and stuffed them, and it turned out that the material he used to stuff the animals was highly laced with asbestos. As a result, I was able to conclude that the abnormal X ray was related to his unusual hobby. The bloody effusion fortunately did not turn out to be malignant and his symptoms were relieved by removal of the fluid.

I also explore any history of upper respiratory symptoms, and problems that relate to the nose, mouth, and throat. Postnasal drip (which your mother called a "stuffy nose") represents an abnormal production of mucus in the upper airways. Usually described by patients as phlegm or mucus in the back of their throat when they wake up in the morning, it can be a clue that there may be equal or greater obstruction in the lower airways.

Another respiratory problem that can be important is a history of nosebleeds. There are many blood vessels in the back of the nose that are particularly fragile and can bleed from a range of problems, including high blood pressure, chronic infection, or polyps. Polyps, which are benign growths, can reflect chronic allergies in the airways. This diagnosis not only is a clue to upper respiratory problems but can alert us to allergic activity elsewhere in the respiratory system.

Sinusitis is frequently a fellow traveler for people with lung disease. It usually begins with pain around the eyes and cheeks and produces a thick discharge from the nose and into the throat. This infection can then migrate to the lower airways, causing serious sinorespiratory problems in the lower airways.

All in the Family

The medical history of your family is critically important. Most chronic lung diseases are not directly inherited, although many tend to run in families. For example, asthma tends to be more frequent in families where allergies of all types are present. We've also seen the form of emphysema which is truly heredi-tary, known as alpha-1 antitrypsin deficiency, it differs from the garden variety emphysema that usually appears in smokers who are over fifty. With alpha-1 antitrypsin, the disease strikes in pa-tients in their thirties and forties.

Strangely enough, it can be often difficult to get a clear idea of the family pulmonary history. When I ask a patient if anyone in their family has diabetes, high blood pressure, heart disease, or cancer, most patients will be able to tell you whether or not these are frequent problems in their family. With pulmonary disease, many people have to think hard and deep about the symptoms, even among their close relatives. They will often need to go home and ask other relatives what they know about the pulmonary history in their family. Chronic cough or short-ness of breath are generally not recognized as signs of serious illness. Death and disabilities are often attributed to heart dis-ease or cancers, and not the underlying lung problems.

Now I have pretty much completed the history, but keep in mind the history never really ends. I will modify that history by what I learn subsequently as I work with you. Just because I have taken the history and moved onto the physical examination and laboratory tests does not mean I forget it. It is always there to guide me. It helps doctors focus on problems that the patient suffers from and allows me to be much smarter than I would be if I just did a physical examination and nothing else.

The Physical Exam

There are findings that relate to the chest that tell me a great deal about how obstructed a patient is. Like most physicians, I start your physical exam at the head and work down to the feet to get an idea of the overall condition. The examination of the eyes, ears, head, nose, and throat can be revealing for a number of reasons. I tap over the sinuses to see if there's any pain that could indicate chronic sinusitis. I look for signs of allergic disease, such as tearing and red eyes, as well as discharge from the nose. Frequently, I look for enlarged lymph nodes up and down the neck (sometimes a sign of an accompanying lung tumor). I feel for an enlarged thyroid, which can influence how tired you may feel.

When it comes to the chest, the examination has four parts. The first is called observation, where I actually look to see how you breathe. I stand behind you to see if you are breathing symmetrically—that is to say, both sides of the thorax are moving equally. I then check to see whether accessory muscles of respiration are being used. Frequently, when somebody has COPD, the configurations of the chest make it difficult to move air in and out of the lungs. When the lungs are hyper-inflated and the diaphragm sags down, most of the breathing is done with the accessory muscles of respiration in the neck.

When we can see these neck muscles being used, the patient appears to be straining to pull his chest up toward his neck. These movements suggest severe airway obstruction.

In severe cases, I can actually see retractions of the chest wall in between the ribs. Normally, when you inhale, there is no movement of the tissue in between the ribs. But when there is severe obstruction with great respiratory distress, that tissue can move inward and give the appearance of collapsing as the person struggles to suck air into the chest.

The second part of the examination is what we call palpation and it consists of putting my hands over your lower back, one on each side of the chest and asking you to say the words "ninety-nine." In healthy lungs, I'll feel a bit of vibration. If there's fluid accumulation in one side of the chest, when a patient says "ninety-nine," I'll feel no vibration because the fluid has damped out the sensation.

The next thing I do is percussion, which is tapping with one finger against the other, up and down the chest. Basically, I look at the lungs as if they were a pair of drums. The lungs are hollow organs filled mainly with air, and as I percuss up and down a healthy chest, I hear a resonant note just as if I were tapping on a snare drum. If the lung is filled with fluid (as in heart failure) or if there's fluid between the lung and the chest wall (as there can be with pleurisy), then the sound I hear is dull rather than a resonant tone.

The last part of the standard examination is to listen to breath sounds with a stethoscope. Normally, over most of the chest, I hear what's called bronchovesicular breath sounds. These are basically the sounds of air moving through the airways as you breathe deeply in and out. You must take a deep breath as you do this or else I will hear virtually nothing. If you breathe normally, only small amounts of air move in and out of the chest and it is very difficult for me to hear anything.

The characteristic thing about bronchovesicular breath sounds is that the inspiratory part of the sound is much longer than the expiratory part. I hear a long *whoosh* during inspiration, but as the patient exhales, it's only a short sound. One pathologic finding is what we call bronchial breath sounds, which is when the sounds of inhaling and exhaling are equal in length. When I hear those over some part of the chest, that usually indicates a sign of consolidation. This implies fluid in the alveoli that could be due to pneumonia, edema, or heart failure.

Other abnormal sounds I listen for are so-called rales, and rhonchi. Rales are dry crackling sounds, usually associated with fluid in the smallest airways. I often hear them in pneumonia and heart failure and they're usually a sign that something abnormal is going on. Rhonchi are wetter sounds. They produce a gurgling noise that usually signifies that there's fluid in larger airways, such as in bronchitis or pneumonia. A third abnormal sound we listen for is wheezing, a high-pitched noise that reflects air moving through a tight airway. In the same way that air through a whistle produces a high-pitched sound, so air moving through a tight airway can produce a squeaky sound. Wheezing is characteristic of anybody who has obstructive lung disease, whether the airways are tight or filled with fluid.

Finally, and perhaps most ominously, there is a finding of the quiet lung. People are naturally very upset when they are told about noisy music box lung with all sorts of sounds, squeaks, whistles, rales, and rattles in it. But probably the most serious of

all sounds is no sound at all. This occurs most commonly in patients who have virtually no lung tissue left. Patients with very
advanced lung disease, either with emphysema or severe
asthma, move so little air in and out of their lungs that I am unable to hear any sounds at all. At this point, these patients are
probably at risk for developing respiratory failure.

The Heart of the Examination

The heart and lungs share the same space in the chest, and we
often find that lung disease is accompanied by some types of
heart disease and vice versa. There is a very specific type of
heart disease known as Cor Pulmonale, which is due to a decline in lung function.

The heart has a right and left side. The right side pumps
blood through the lungs and the left side pumps blood through
the rest of the body, the main organs and the muscles. When
the lungs become sick and damaged, the heart has a great deal
of difficulty pumping blood through the blood vessels that go
through the lungs. This causes a backup of fluid in the right
heart, producing right-sided heart failure. The muscles of the
right heart are normally much weaker than the muscles of
the left heart. One of the results of right heart failure is that the
jugular veins in the neck swell, particularly when the patient is
seated or semireclining. The blood backs up into other organs
of the body. For example, the liver becomes enlarged, and
painfully congested. There is also backup of fluid into the
lower parts of the body and the legs become swollen with
edema.

To evaluate the impact of lung disease on the heart, as well as to discover other types of heart disease that could impact on lung function, I do a cardiac examination, which, like the examination of the chest, consists of four parts.

I look at the chest to see if I can actually see the heart beating against the chest wall. Normally, there's a little heave in the area of the left side of the chest where the heart has its maximum impulse. When the heart is abnormal, for example, if there is a right-sided heart failure, the heave is more toward the right and may actually be seen. This gives me a clue that the right side of the heart is struggling. I feel the point of maximum impulse of the heart and we can make sure there are no abnormal sounds. I percuss the heart just as I did with the lungs, again, to get an idea of its size. When the heart becomes very enlarged, the border of the heart moves out toward the left or toward the right side of the chest.

I listen to the heart with a stethoscope and note abnormal sounds. My cardiologist colleagues tell me there are up to sixteen different heart sounds you can hear with each beat of the heart, but most mortal physicians hear at most four. These sounds correspond to the opening and closing of the valves inside the heart. Normally, there is silence between the sounds.

Sometimes, when there is a narrowing of the passageway between the chambers of the heart or in the blood vessels leaving the heart, I hear what is called a murmur. This sound represents a turbulence in blood flow in the heart or blood vessels, just as a wheeze represents turbulent airflow through an airway. A murmur may be the result of some normal or abnormal variations in the heart. Many murmurs are just what we call physiologic (or nonpathologic), while others can signify disease. I also listen for the rhythm of the heart. The normal resting heart rate is regular and runs between 60 and 100 beats per minute. Anything faster is known as tachycardia and anything slower is called bradycardia.

I examine the abdomen because signs of right heart failure that go along with very severe lung disease can first appear as an enlarged liver. I look at the extremities and legs, checking for edema or a difference in size between the two that might indicate a blocked or poorly functioning vein. I palpitate the arteries that run along the legs to see if the pulses are normal. Then I take your blood pressure and count the number of breaths you take each minute.

By this time, I have a pretty good idea of a probable diagnosis. For most patients who are suspected of having lung disease, the most important next step is a chest X ray. For nearly 100 years, the chest X ray has been the cornerstone of a pulmonary workup, and even in our digital age, the simple X ray is still an important screening tool. When normal, the chest X ray provides a great deal of information. A chest X ray that is abnormal provides equally valuable and different information. There are many lung diseases, such as asthma and bronchitis, that will usually have absolutely normal chest X rays. By contrast, lung cancer, severe emphysema, and hyperinflation may all be picked up on a simple chest X ray.

Testing for Strength and Weakness

The next step is to expand our findings of the physical examination with laboratory tests. I usually start with a series of tests that provides insight in different types of lung function.

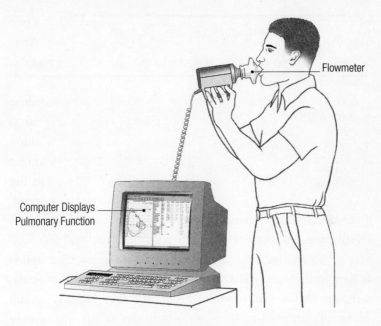

Flowmeter

Computer Displays
Pulmonary Function

The spirometry test provides a physician with a clear profile
of your lung function.

The workhorse of pulmonary function tests uses a machine called a spirometer. The patient blows into a mouthpiece attached to a pneumotach, a device that measures airflow. This measuring device is connected to a computer programmed to convert the flow signal into volume measurements. The results are printed out in the form of numbers and graphs. Before testing, I enter your vital statistics—age, weight, height, race, and sex—into the computer. This provides me with a predicted set of results for these characteristics. This test gives us a series of at least three to four measurements, which when taken together provide me with a better understanding of the causes of your symptoms.

Pulmonary Function Printout

Index	Unit	Meas.✓	Pred.*	% Pred
FVC	Liters	2.91	2.97	98
FEV1	Liters	2.37	2.43	98
FEV1/FVC%		81.4	81.4	100
PEF	Liters/second	5.6	5.8	97%
Forced Expiratory Time: 6.2 seconds				

*Predicted
✓Measured

The first measurement is called forced vital capacity, or FVC. Placing the mouthpiece between your lips, you will inhale as deeply as you can, hold your breath for a moment, then exhale as hard and fast as you can for at least six seconds. This measurement is the total volume of air that the lung can exhale when fully inflated and it gives me an idea of the size of your lung.

The second number that is measured is the FEV1, the amount of air in liters that can be blown out in the first second of this test. This gives me an idea of the ability of your lung to move air in and out quickly. For example, in emphysema, the lungs can usually inhale normally, producing a normal FVC. But when patients with emphysema try to exhale, the airways collapse and the lungs cannot empty rapidly so that the FEV1 is reduced.

The third number that we get is the FEV1/FVC ratio, which is the amount of air that can be exhaled in one second expressed as a fraction of FVC. This is important because it gives me an idea of the degree of obstruction in the lungs. As obstructive lung disease progresses, patients are unable to fully exhale rapidly and I can measure the progression of this problem with this ratio.

The fourth number that we get from this single test is the peak expiratory flow, known as PEF, which is the maximum speed at which the air is blown out. I repeat the spirometry tests three times in a row, checking to see if all the results are within 5 percent of one another.

Home Care That You Can Measure

Peak expiratory flow (PEF) is particularly useful because it can be measured with inexpensive home devices. We often give handheld peak flow meters to asthma patients to monitor serial changes in lung function, thereby picking up problems that develop long before there are any changes in symptoms. The peak flow meter can measure the degree of bronchial constriction and serve as a warning system of an impending attack. When the peak flow meter readings drop significantly, patients are instructed to increase medications and immediately call a physician.

Testing the Results

Once I have a good idea of the basic pulmonary function, I want to see how your lungs react to bronchodilators—a class of drugs that open airways for easier breathing. The results may give me a better idea of the causes behind symptoms. You will take two puffs of a short-acting inhaler, then we wait for ten minutes for the drug to take effect. Then the spirometry test is repeated. If you have asthma, I will see an improvement of at least 12 percent in the FEV1. If the response is less than 12 percent, the problem may be overinflation of the lungs, as seen in emphysema or chronic bronchitis.

Even in the face of a negative response to bronchodilators, I often still prescribe a trial of these drugs. A single test may not indicate what happens over several weeks of treatment. A slight cold or previous medication may also affect test results accuracy.

Challenging the Results

In some cases, I will test the degree of airway sensitivity with a bronchoconstrictor, a substance that triggers airways to narrow. Usually, I use methacholine, a chemical related to acetyl-choline, the mediator that controls the tone of the smooth muscle in the airways.

Individuals with asthma are exquisitely sensitive to the con-strictive effects of methacholine. For example, a healthy person can breathe in an aerosol solution of methacholine containing at least 10 mg/cc with hardly a response. Asthmatic lungs may respond to quantities as low as .1 mg or less.

To do this test, you will inhale five breaths of an aerosol containing a known amount of methacholine. I will measure spirometry before and after the challenge. I usually start with just plain water and then increase the concentrations of metha-choline until I see a response in your spirometry—usually a 10 percent or more fall in FEV1. This test is generally considered safe. However, some very sensitive individuals may develop a very severe full-blown asthma attack following the procedure.

Methacholine tests are a useful tool for establishing a diagno-sis of asthma when there are a number of other health issues to be evaluated. It can be helpful when patients have symptoms that might be due to chronic sinusitis or reflux. Recently, methacholine challenge tests have been used at Mt. Sinai to evaluate the lung function of rescue workers involved with the collapse of the World Trade Center in New York.

Spirometry tests are the foundation of the pulmonary workup. Painless, quick, and inexpensive, I believe that spirometry should be part of an annual physical for all former and current smokers. I feel it can pick up problems long before they cause symptoms, permanent lung remodeling, and loss of pulmonary function. I am delighted to see that more internists and family physicians are including spirometry in their routine examinations.

The Diffusion Capacity Test

I often want to measure how well your lungs can transfer oxygen from the air into the blood, so I will order a diffusion capacity test. During this test, you will inhale extremely low concentrations of carbon monoxide mixed with helium, oxygen, and nitrogen and hold your breath for a short period of time. When you exhale into the tube attached to a machine, the flow and volume of your breath as well as its carbon monoxide and helium concentrations will be measured. This provides an idea of how easy (or how difficult) it is for your lungs to transfer gases from inhaled air into the blood. When emphysema is present, the alveoli, the lung structures responsible for gas exchange in the lungs, are damaged and we see a decline in the diffusing capacity. This gives me an idea of the severity of the damage to the airways. By contrast, in asthma, diffusing capacity is usually not affected and this test helps me distinguish between the different types of COPD, even when symptoms are very similar.

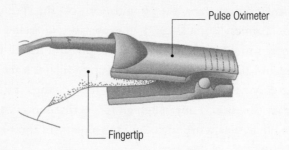

By shining a light through the finger, the pulse oximeter can measure the amount of oxygen transported by the blood.

The Pulse Oximetry Test

In this test, we attach a finger monitor called a pulse oximeter (the shortened form is pulse ox) that shines a light on the skin which allows us to determine the oxygen saturation of the hemoglobin in your blood. Here's how it works: each hemoglobin molecule can hold four molecules of oxygen. As more oxygen comes into the blood, more of the hemoglobin oxygen attachment sites become filled. Since your blood contains a fixed amount of hemoglobin (15 grams per 100 cc's of blood in a healthy person), if enough oxygen gets in the blood, it saturates all or nearly all of the receptors. The color of the blood changes with its saturation and this is what we measure.

Oxygen saturation is expressed as a percentage. Most healthy people have a saturation that ranges between 95 and 100 percent and in a healthy cardiopulmonary system that number does not change with exercise. When there are pulmonary problems, exercise will produce a significant drop in oxygen saturation. Oxygen saturation below 90 percent will cause a significant strain on heart and lungs. As lung disease progresses, oxygen saturation can fall below 90 percent, even when the person is at rest.

If there is still any ambiguity about the nature or extent of your lung problem, I will often order an additional test to measure your residual lung volume. This is the amount of air that remains in the lung after you have exhaled all the air that you can. In COPD, residual volume tends to increase as the lung traps air. The result? A lung that is one and a half to two

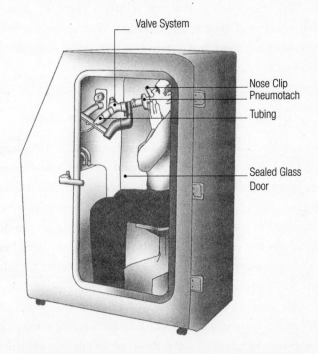

Looking like a combination phone booth and minisubmarine, the body plethysmograph measures the size of the lung as well as airway resistance. Because the lung is frequently enlarged and airway resistance is increased in COPD, we can use this test to confirm a diagnosis.

times its normal volume. I have found that the best way to gather this important measurement is with a *plethysmograph,* a machine that resembles an old-fashioned telephone booth.

For this test, you will sit on a low stool in a tightly sealed chamber and breathe quietly through a mouthpiece. When you feel comfortable, the mouthpiece is blocked and then you pant against the closed air tube. This maneuver measures the amount of compressible gas within the lung, and it is an effective way to distinguish between obstructive and restrictive lung disease. For example, in patients with early emphysema, the residual volume of air left in the lung is large, whereas in pulmonary scarring (which is a form of restrictive lung disease), the residual volume is reduced.

Computed Axial Tomography (CAT) Scan

CAT scans are increasingly used in the diagnosis of lung disease. A CAT scan is a series of X rays taken with a machine that moves up and down your body and converts the information of the X rays into a three-dimensional image. The results are usually displayed as a series of horizontal "cuts" through the body, which allows me to visualize the lungs as a loaf of sliced bread. This configuration allows me to examine the normal and abnormal structures at each level of the lung, visualizing the three-dimensional configurations within the chest.

CAT scans are particularly effective for finding areas of emphysema. In patients who have this type of chronic obstructive lung disease, the lung is literally eaten away, and we are now able to find signs of this damage at a much earlier stage with CAT scans. This type of destruction starts out as a patchy disease, and as the disease progresses, the areas of destruction coalesce. Eventually, when the damage is widespread, they become apparent on a chest X ray. CAT scans can pick up this damage far earlier and give me a much better opportunity to evaluate and treat the damage at an early stage.

CAT scans are now being used to screen for lung cancers. I am able to see spots in the lungs when they are a fraction of the size of those that were visible with a simple chest X ray. In the past, nodules in the lungs less than two or three centimeters were very difficult to pick up on the routine X ray. With a CAT scan, we can find nodules that are one or two millimeters, ten to twenty times smaller than nodules that would be visible on an X ray. The downside of these findings is that not all of these nodules are lung cancers. They are frequently little areas of scar tissue from infections and doctors are not always sure how to approach these findings. For the majority of patients, I recommend that very small spots be followed periodically over a period of two years. If there is no change, I am comfortable that it is just a benign blip on the X ray.

A Drop of Blood

The standard blood tests for your pulmonary workup include complete blood count, BUN (blood urea nitrogen), electrolytes, and liver function tests. These tests are done just to gauge the general health to make sure there are no other diseases or abnormalities that are complicating the situation.

But there are some specific facts you and I can learn from these tests. For example, if your white blood cell count is elevated, it usually indicates there's some sort of inflammation or infection. I also look for levels of a particular type of white blood cells called eosinophils. Normally, they represent less than 5 percent of all white blood cells that circulate in the blood. When this count is elevated, it may be a sign of allergy, possibly related to asthma. It helps me to characterize the cause of your symptoms and provides a scale to measure the value of our treatment plan.

We can also do specialized tests to gauge your level of allergy antibodies. Generally, we do what is called an IgE test. IgE is the antibody that is responsible for a number of common allergies. The normal level of IgE usually is 100 International Units (IU) or less. In allergy, it can be elevated to several hundred or even 1,000 units. Having a normal IgE does not necessarily mean that you are allergy-free. If I still suspect specific allergies, I order an antibody series known as radio-allergoabsorbent or RAST tests. This blood test measures the individual IgE levels RELATIVE to different allergens. I test for common culprits, including dust mites, cockroaches, different types of local pollen, and sensitivity to both dog and cat dander.

When it is appropriate, the blood test can also measure for the hereditary form of emphysema. The most commonly used test measures the level of alpha-1 antitrypsin in the blood. This is the compound that protects against destruction of normal elastin in the lungs. If this test is positive, we can follow up with a genetic profiling test to determine risks among family members for this type of inherited emphysema.

If warranted, I also will do a test for cystic fibrosis, a hereditary disease that involves the lungs, causing repeated infections and progressive lung damage. This is usually a disease of young children, but doctors now realize that nearly one quarter of individuals with the disease are not diagnosed until their teens and twenties. During the Vietnam War when I was a physician in the Navy, I saw a young patient with severe pneumonia. Alex was barely eighteen, five feet tall, with very thin, fragile, white-blond hair. It turned out that the underlying cause of his lung problem was not an infection but undiagnosed cystic fibrosis. In hindsight, Alex had more than his share of childhood health problems. He had frequent upper respiratory infections and digestive malabsorption problems so severe that it stunted his growth. His brittle, thin hair was actually a sign of malnutrition, which happens with the malabsorption cycle frequent in cystic fibrosis. Alex had frequent respiratory infections, but was just not diagnosed until he developed significant lung problems. In a young patient with unusual signs and severe symptoms, I may do a test for cystic fibrosis, just to rule out this possibility.

Testing for Damage

When I need to evaluate you for pulmonary disability, I may do an exercise test, which is a simple method for determining the impairment of the cardiopulmonary system. We use a bicycle or a treadmill to measure different factors, including how much oxygen is inhaled and how much CO_2 is exhaled during exercise, as well as heart rate and blood pressure. These measurements will give me an idea of how limited you may be by your lung disease and how much work you actually can do. I can also do these tests to distinguish between heart problems (which can also cause shortness of breath) and lung disease.

Often we can judge how much of your disability is due to the lung disease and how much is due to cardiac problems.

The Humane Use of Nuclear Power

I can use a variety of nuclear scans to get a better idea of the progression of lung disease. The most common scan that I order is the ventilation perfusion scan that looks simultaneously at how breathing and circulation in the lungs interact. This test is particularly helpful in picking up blood clots in the lung. It also tells me about regional areas in the lung, how well they are working or not working. Frequently, patients who have to undergo lung surgery will need these tests to anticipate benefit of the surgery or complications that may occur.

I have recently begun using Positron Electron Tomography (PET) scan. This test can be useful in telling me the difference between a cancer nodule and one that is just simply scar tissue or a benign lung shadow. It also can pick up areas of spreading cancer.

If the condition warrants it, I do a gallium scan, which is helpful for patients who have interstitial lung disease. When the disease is active, the gallium is taken up by the irritated white blood cells and "lights up" the lung and other affected tissues, indicating areas of infection or inflammation.

It is important to remember that it is possible for you to have more than one lung disease at the same time and may need different treatment plans of frequent strategies, in order to resolve each of the problems. I tend to use these more sophisticated tests when patients who are not responding to traditional treatment or whose symptoms suddenly get worse fail to respond to approaches that have worked in the past.

Now that we have a firm diagnosis, I am ready to start to develop an effective treatment plan. But before I start prescribing medication, I want to work with you on the lifestyle factors that affect your health. We'll start exploring the role of diet in pulmonary problems in the next chapter.

Chapter 6

Eat Right, Breathe Easy

"I hate it when patients ask me what they should eat. It makes me feel like a waiter," grumbled the attending physician "as we made rounds at the old Victorian hospital. In my last year in medical school in the late 1960s, I went to England for a two-month rotation at Queen's Square Hospital in London. The silver-haired Harley Street doctor who led the ward rounds that morning was a physician of the old school. Supremely confident, and almost imperious, he felt that his presence at the bedside was all a patient would need or should expect. Medical questions were answered in formal, distant tones. Nutritional questions were usually answered with a pat on the shoulder and vague advice to "go easy on puddings."

In the United States, we were already concerned about the impact of diet on health and longevity, but in Great Britain, the concept was not yet on the radar of older physicians. Perhaps the memory of food rationing was still too recent to think that food could play a role in disease. In fact, the National Health

Service urged people to eat more eggs with the slogan: "Go to work on an egg."

Over the past forty years, research both here and abroad has demonstrated extensive links between nutrition and heart disease, hypertension, and even certain types of cancer. More recently, doctors have begun to look for the same type of causal relationship between diet and chronic lung disease.

There is an intriguing molecular basis for this research. As we've seen, it is known that oxidative stress, the impact of high levels of free radicals is part of the pathologic process of asthma and COPD. We also know that dietary factors, such as vitamins, prevent or reverse free radical activity. Vitamins C, E, and beta carotene are all antioxidants and in theory could shield the respiratory system from oxidative damage from air pollution and cigarettes. Vitamin C is a free radical scavenger that operates both inside and outside of the cells in the lung. Its companion, vitamin E, can be found both in the lung fluid and within the lipid membranes of the lung cells, working to transform oxygen free radicals and lipid peroxyl free radicals, some of the lung's most destructive species, to less dangerous molecules. Beta carotene, the form of vitamin A found in fruits and vegetables, can be found in lung tissue membranes. The different locations and activities of each of these vitamins could provide a wide range of antioxidant protection for the respiratory system.

A number of well-designed studies have demonstrated this may well be true. In the Seven Countries Study that looked at the nutrition and health patterns in seven Western nations, we found that where the diet was high in fruits and vegetables, the incidence of COPD was significantly lower, even in people who smoked cigarettes. When COPD was present, it was less severe, produced fewer symptoms, and had lower mortality rates.

The Second National Health and Nutrition Examination Survey, known as NHANES II, looked at health and diet patterns of 9,000 adults in the United States. Researchers found that people with low vitamin C blood levels had a higher incidence of bronchitis. Researchers from the University of Nottingham reported similar findings. Following 2,600 current and former smokers, the doctors found that persons eating just five apples or three tomatoes each week had better lung function and less asthma. A particularly encouraging study from England recently reported that even people who smoked a pack of cigarettes a day could benefit from a vegetable rich diet. A researcher from the University of Southampton found that just a tablespoon of vegetables per day cut the risk of developing COPD by almost 50 percent. A study carried out in China found specifically that vitamin C seemed to offer pulmonary protection. Three thousand men and women underwent pulmonary function tests, and their blood was analyzed for vitamin levels. After adjusting the data for age and smoking habits, researchers found a direct correlation between vitamin C levels and pulmonary function measurements. That is to say, pulmonary function was better in people with high levels of vitamin C.

Given that vitamin C is one of the trinity of antioxidant all-stars, these findings were exciting but not really surprising. Vitamin C, also known as ascorbic acid, is a water-soluble vitamin that traps free radicals, preventing lipid peroxidation. This means that fats do not change forms, which increases arterial blockage. In addition, it has been suggested that vitamin C may repair lung tissue damage through collagen synthesis. Others believe that it may modify prostaglandin production, another mediator that provokes asthma-related inflammation. Some experts theorize that vitamin C may prevent the overdestruction of elastin fibers.

Found in citrus fruits, tomatoes, and strawberries, vitamin C is important for healthy gums, collagen growth, and wound healing. Vitamin C protects healthy cells from free radical damage, possibly inhibiting the proliferation of cancerous cells. Some studies suggest that vitamin C may block the conversion of nitrates and nitrites into cancer-causing compounds and may theoretically reduce the risk for certain types of cancer. The recommended daily allowance for vitamin C is 60 mg/day, an amount that can be met by a cup of strawberries. Larger doses of vitamin C are usually not toxic but may cause digestive distress due to its acidity. The body cannot store vitamin C and needs a fresh supply every day. A diet low in vitamin C has been linked to lowered immunity and bleeding gums, features of the vitamin deficiency known as scurvy.

A Vitamin for Healthy Lungs

A study out of Johns Hopkins found a statistically significant relationship between the incidence of airway obstruction and the decreasing levels of all forms of vitamin A. Reports showed that men whose diets were low in vitamin A rich foods, such as tomatoes, sweet potatoes, and spinach, had a higher incidence of chronic lung problems, including bronchitis and decreased lung function.

Vitamin A is a fat-soluble vitamin that is crucial for the development of epithelial tissue in the skin, eyes, and the lungs. A powerful antioxidant, vitamin A protects the body from the oxidative stress caused by pollution, cigarette smoke, and sunlight. Studies have shown that the antioxidant activity of vitamin A and beta carotene is linked to lower risk of heart disease and some types of cancers.

Vitamin A is found in fish oil, liver, milk, and cheese, but the majority of this vitamin in our diet comes from plant sources. Dark green and yellow vegetables, such as spinach and sweet potatoes, contain beta carotene that is converted into vitamin A in the body.

Lack of vitamin A can cause vision problems, such as night blindness, but that condition is very rare in this country. A hardy compound, it stays active even after cooking, canning, and even drying. The recommended daily allowance is 2,300 IU for women and 3,000 IU for men, which can be met with one wedge of cantaloupe or one third cup of cooked spinach. Since it is a fat-soluble nutrient, the body can store this vitamin and excessive supplementation can be toxic. High levels of vitamin A can cause dry itchy skin, abnormal hair growth, water retention, bone pain, and possibly birth defects. For this reason, most physicians do not recommend vitamin A supplements. You can get all the vitamin A you need in a diet rich in fruits and vegetables and will thereby avoid problems caused by the high dosages found in some pills.

Different Forms of Vitamin A

A form of vitamin A known as retinoic acid has been shown to restore normal growth patterns of epithelial cells. In skin care formulations, retinoic acid (also known as Retin A) can reverse signs of skin aging by stimulating the growth of elastin and collagen fibers. Now a husband-and-wife research team from Georgetown University School of Medicine have discovered that a related form of retinoic acid promotes the regrowth of new healthy alveoli in laboratory animals. Gloria and Donald Massaro suggested that the retinoids may modify antielastase enzymes, reducing inflammation, and allowing the body to heal and rebuild. The success of the animal studies was so promising that it quickly led to a five center nationwide study sponsored by the NIH. The goal of this study is to see if retinoic acid can repair and regrow alveoli in people suffering from emphysema.

The King of the Antioxidants

A study published in the *American Journal of Respiratory and Critical Care Medicine* found that dietary intake of vitamin E could improve lung function in older people. The Third National Health and Nutrition Examination Survey (NHANES III) found that vitamin E intake had a positive correlation with lung function tests. In other words, people with an adequate vitamin E intake had higher FEV1 results.

Often called the king of the antioxidants, vitamin E has been linked to a reduction in risk of heart disease and strokes. It appears that vitamin E may prevent the oxidation of Low-Density Lipoprotein (LDL) cholesterol. Why is that important? There are two primary forms of cholesterol—the "good"

High-Density Lipoprotein (HDL) cholesterol and the "bad" LDL cholesterol. We have long recognized that elevated LDL cholesterol is associated with an increased risk of coronary heart disease. Doctors now believe that LDL cholesterol is not inherently bad. It is only when it becomes oxidized (such as by free radicals) that it becomes a threat to the circulatory system. Oxidized LDL cholesterol produces an inflammatory reaction in the walls of the arteries. LDL cholesterol piles up at the site of inflammation, which leads to an artery-obstructing plaque that can cause a heart attack or stroke. Research now indicates that Vitamin E may prevent oxidation of LDL and can keep arteries open and healthy. The RDA for Vitamin E is 30 IU. The best food sources for this important antioxidant include vegetable oils, wheat germ, olives, and nuts.

The Brilliant Color of Health

We have only recently become aware of thousands of substances known as phytochemicals or bioflavonoids, which are natural ingredients in a wide range of fruits and vegetables. For plants, these chemicals provide protection against bacteria, fungi, and insects. We are now recognizing that bioflavonoids may have disease-fighting properties for human health. For example, the bioflavonoid quercetin found in wine is believed to be the answer behind the "French Paradox."

Although Gallic meals feature butter, pâté, and the eponymous french fries, the French enjoy an enviously low rate of heart disease. Doctors believe that it is the antioxidant properties in quercetin-rich red wine that provides this cardioprotection. One study found that just one glass of wine with lunch and/or dinner prevented oxidation of LDL cholesterol, which if unchecked could lead to plaque buildup in the arteries.

The Zutphyn study from Holland suggested that the quercetin didn't have to come from wine. The five-year Dutch study followed a group of 100 older men whose diets included quercetin rich foods, such as green apples, onions, and green tea. The result? At the end of the study, these men had a significantly reduced mortality rate, compared to those whose diets were low in quercetin. In addition, they had lower rates of both asthma and COPD, suggesting that quercetin offered pulmonary protective benefits.

Lycopene is another bioflavonoid that gives tomatoes their glorious color. A study from Italy found that men who consumed seven or more servings a week of tomatoes had a 50 percent reduced risk of gastric cancer compared to men who ate less than two servings of tomatoes weekly. A new study from the State University of Buffalo suggests that bioflavonoids like lycopene can have an impact on pulmonary health. The research looked at more than 1,600 healthy people ages thirty-five to seventy-nine in western New York. After adjusting for age and smoking history, researchers found that those with the lowest levels of antioxidants (including lycopene, beta carotene, lutein, and retinol) had consistently lower pulmonary function numbers. As the levels of antioxidants rose, so did pulmonary function.

Lycopene research from Israel is equally promising for asthma. Twenty people with exercise-induced asthma were treated with 30 mg of lycopene supplement/day. After four weeks, more than half were able to exercise without developing wheezing or coughing.

The Role of Diet in Asthma

Nutritional status also seems to play an equally important role in the development and severity of asthma. Particular attention has been paid to the role of omega-3 fatty acids found in fish. Studies from Australia have shown that children who ate fish more than once a week were 30 to 70 percent less likely to have asthma than children who ate fish less often.

These observations mirror findings of adult epidemiological studies. It is believed that the very low levels of asthma in Greenland Eskimos and in Mediterranean countries is related to the importance that fish plays in their diet. Fish oil acts to inhibit transformation of arachidonic acid into leukotrienes, which are important mediators of asthma bronchoconstriction. While fish oils may reduce the frequency of asthma symptoms, polyunsaturated oils may increase pulmonary problems. In a study funded by the British Lung Foundation, doctors found that adults with asthma consumed more polyunsaturated fats than an equivalent group with no history of wheezing.

On a molecular level, these findings make a great deal of sense. Oxidative stress, the result of high levels of free radicals and the inflammatory factors they provoke, is a well-defined trigger in both asthma and COPD. Each day air pollution, allergens, and cigarette smoke subject the body to waves of problem-causing free radicals. In laboratory animals, antioxidants have been shown to offer protection against harmful pollution. Rats fed a diet low in vitamin C and E sustained more damage from ozone than those maintained on standard laboratory feed. Antioxidants like vitamin A, C, and E, as well as omega-3 fatty acids, have been shown to prevent and reverse free radical formation and reduce oxidative stress. The population studies that supported these theories led doctors to the logical next step . . . with disappointing results.

The Slip Between the Lab and the Lip

A joint study from the National Public Health Institute in Finland and the National Cancer Institute in Bethesda, Maryland, followed the health status of almost 30,000 male smokers. In a well-designed study, the men were given different combinations of vitamin supplements and were carefully followed for an average of six years. At regular intervals, subjects were interviewed and given complete and thorough examinations. Despite exhaustive statistical analysis, no differences were found between the men who received vitamin supplements and those that didn't. In other words, the vitamin supplements had no impact on the pulmonary health.

A study published in the British medical journal *Thorax* found that fish supplements had provided no change in symptoms in cases of mild asthma. Even more troubling were the results from the Beta Carotene and Retinol Efficiency Study (CARET) that followed 18,000 people at risk for lung cancer. They were given beta carotene supplements and at the end of three years researchers were shocked to find a 40 percent **increase** in lung cancer mortality in subjects taking the high dose supplements. Equally frightening was the fact that subjects in the CARET study showed a 30 percent increase in mortality from all causes, including heart disease.

What Went Wrong?

The results were both surprising and troubling. Not only did vitamin supplements fail to secure health benefits, they actually were associated with increased lung cancer and heart disease death rates. There were numerous reasons suggested for these findings. Some believed the dosage of supplements was either too high or too low. Others suggested that the studies were done on people whose lungs were past help and that antioxidants needed to be given for years before symptoms began to be effective. Others suggested that the length of these supplement studies was too short and more years of treatment were needed before benefits could be seen.

It has also been suggested that perhaps the ratio of nutrients as they appear naturally in foods are an important part of disease prevention. Additionally, rather than vitamins, there can be as yet unrecognized compounds in foods that are actually the source of decreased pulmonary risk.

What Do These Studies Mean?

Despite definitive evidence of their efficacy in deficiency situations, the role of vitamins in lung disease is a frequent concern of my patients and one of the key questions most frequently asked by them. For example, early one morning as I was making rounds, I stopped by the bedside of one of my longtime patients with COPD. Barbara had been admitted over the weekend for respiratory failure. After a few days of oxygen, steroids, and antibiotics, she was much better. When I entered her room, I was delighted to see her sitting up and eating breakfast. As soon as she saw me, Barbara reached into the drawer of her bedside table and pulled out a page-long list. "It was so difficult to remember what I was taking when the ambulance brought me in," she explained. "Can you check this and see if I got it all down?"

The single-column list covered an entire page and included the complete alphabet of vitamins, an assortment of Chinese herbs, enzymes, amino acids—even a few items that were completely new to me. Then at the bottom were the five medications I had prescribed.

It was not the first time I had seen such a list. Until recently, I have taken a fairly benign view of nutritional supplements. Although I recommended taking one or maybe even two multivitamins each day for nutritional backup, I didn't try to argue against so-called nutriceuticals. There was enough interesting laboratory and epidemiological structure to leave at least a rationale for taking additional antioxidants.

Then came those supplemental clinical trials which actually showed an increase in cancer rates in patients receiving supplements. Researchers examining the failures of these trials noted that high doses of vitamins can actually *promote* free radicals production, possibly producing a state of oxidative stress.

The troubling findings have led me to change my laid-back attitude to supplements. I now urge my patients to get their antioxidants in the way they have shown to be effective—in a diet rich in fruits and vegetables.

At this point, all we know with any certainty is that it is the dietary patterns which offer protection, not isolated supplementation. As a physician, I need to provide my patients with nutritional information that has been shown to be both safe and effective, and with that standard, we need to take our cues within the best available dietary evidence. Today we see that the benefits are in the diet and not in a pill. But what does that mean in terms of practical daily meal plans?

Diet and the Hippocratic Oath

First do no harm. This is the first rule of the physician and one that I feel physicians should keep in mind when offering nutritional counseling. Bad nutritional advice is no longer a victimless crime. Over the past four decades, we've gleaned new knowledge that links nutrition to disease and has led us to make many different recommendations, a number of which we are now wishing we had never made and are now reversing.

For example, when we first recognized the role that diet plays in heart disease, we believed that it was the fully formed cholesterol found in eggs, butter, and other high-fat dairy products that caused problems. Our first recommendations were to eliminate these foods, and we were very disappointed to find that the heart disease rates were not declining. What we didn't know at the time was that it was the saturated fats in meats that were then formed into cholesterol in our body, and without restricting these foods, we would not see any change in cholesterol levels.

We were equally misled when we decided that polyunsaturated fats were the answer. By looking at the health patterns and diets in China and Japan, where there are high levels of polyunsaturated fats in the diets, primarily in the oils used for cooking such as peanut oil, we felt that they offered protection against heart disease, and so we urged people to use margarine and corn oil rather than butter, and to use foods made with polyunsaturated oils.

The problem was that polyunsaturates were themselves then linked to higher rates of certain types of cancers. Even worse, when polyunsaturates were used in food processing and production, they changed to transfatty acids that not only were now linked to an increased risk of cancer, but actually raised the cholesterol levels.

More recently, we began advocating soy and soy proteins to lower cholesterol, as well as decrease the risk of certain types of cancers. Based on the low rates of breast cancer in Japanese women who had a high soy intake, we advocated including soy in our meals to capture these benefits. Even the normally conservative Food and Drug Administration (FDA) allowed packaged and processed foods to make claims for cholesterol lowering in products that contained at least twenty-five grams of soy. Now new studies report a disturbing link between increased risk of estrogen-based breast and uterine tumors with higher intake of soy.

The Pulmonary Protective Diet

When I broach the idea of diet to keep pulmonary symptoms under control, my patients look concerned. When I explain that my focus is on the adequate intake of foods that apparently lower pulmonary risk, as well as reduce the risk of heart disease, they are happy that I am not suggesting yet another restricted diet that makes it difficult to eat with friends and family.

The healthiest and safest diets need to include a wide range of foods to ensure you receive the best of all nutrients. There are only a few foods that should be restricted or prohibited, and it's even possible on this diet to put together meals in fast-food restaurants, coffee shops, and diners. Known as the DASH diet, it was originally introduced by the NIH to lower blood pressure and cardiac risks. We have studied the results of this diet for over the last ten years, and the numbers just keep getting better.

DASH stands for Dietary Approaches to Stop Hypertension. Use of this diet proved that elevated blood pressure can be reduced with an eating plan that is low in saturated fat, total fat, and cholesterol, and rich in fruits, vegetables, fiber, and low-fat dairy foods. The plan is rich in magnesium, potassium, calcium, protein, and fiber. This successful diet started with the same types of observations that we are making now when we look at pulmonary problems.

Epidemiologically, scientists saw that people whose diets were low in sodium had reduced levels of hypertension; similarly, they found that in people whose diets were low in calcium and/or magnesium, the blood pressure was elevated. But when they tried to correct blood pressure by simply adding these minerals as supplements, the results were disappointing. There was just no improvement. Instead of simply adding nutrient supplements to the standard American diet, they decided to design a program that naturally reflected the eating pattern associated with lower blood pressure rates. The results were dramatic. In fact, blood pressure reduction started within two weeks of beginning the DASH diet. The longer people are on it, the more blood pressure headed toward normal. More recently, the DASH-II diet results were just released, which showed even better results were obtained when this fiber-and-nutrient-rich diet was coupled with a sharp reduction in sodium values. Both clinical studies that looked at individual patients and epidemiological studies, which analyzed large populations, have shown that high sodium levels in the diet can affect lung problems, making this diet doubly beneficial for people with pulmonary problems.

The DASH diet looks very much like a typical American diet that has been adjusted or tweaked. What is particularly important is that you get in those five to seven servings of fruits and vegetables every day, as well as generous servings of whole grains and low-fat dairy products to cover the nutritional landscape.

No diet that is too strange or demanding, no matter how intelligently and scientifically it is designed, will succeed for a simple reason: few people will be able to follow it. By contrast, the DASH diet can be followed easily wherever you go, both at home and in restaurants. The DASH diet is not expensive. It is affordable and it doesn't need elaborate cooking or exotic ingredients. The foods are available at every supermarket throughout the world. I think the only place that you might have trouble following the DASH diet is in the air, if all they serve on a plane are pretzels and beverages.

Close-Up: The DASH Program

The basic DASH diet is formulated on a 2,000 calorie a day intake. This is good for the average-sized man but might be somewhat too heavy a calorie load for a woman. For the average woman, you can lower the calorie intake to 1,500 to 1,800 calories a day. Let's look at each component in depth to understand the benefits they offer.

The DASH diet recommends seven to eight servings of grain and grain products a day, but for a woman you can reduce this to four to five servings. It's important to understand what a serving is. A serving of carbohydrate is one slice of bread or a scant half a cup of rice, pasta, and cereal. Clearly, this is a smaller-sized serving than you get in most restaurants. One rainy day when we ordered Chinese takeout, I decided to just see how many servings of rice there were in the typical container of vegetable fried rice. I stopped counting when I reached seven half a cup servings. The size of the portions of all foods need to be counted, or the calorie intake will be very high.

Grains and grain products are marvelous sources of B vitamins, fiber, and vitamin E. For optimum health, look for whole grain products, such as whole wheat breads, English muffins, pita breads, cereals, and slow-cooked oatmeal. Always look for unsalted or unsweetened cereals. You can have a cereal for breakfast, sandwich for lunch, and a potato for dinner, and not only feel comfortable and full, but know that you are providing the nutrition your body needs.

There should be four to five servings of vegetables a day, and servings do not have to be huge. Try to have as much variety of vegetables as possible to get the maximum number of different types of nutrients and bioflavonoids. For example, dark green lettuce leaves are high in vitamin C and beta carotene, while tomatoes are rich in a bioflavonoid called lycopene, which is linked to lower cancer rates, better eyesight, and lower risk of prostate cancer. If you add lettuce, tomato, and onion to every sandwich, you're getting a wonderful smorgasbord of antioxidants in a small sandwich. Keep in mind that different antioxidants act on different free radicals and a varied diet will provide the broadest antioxidant protection.

You have almost an infinite choice of vegetables, depending on your taste and the season. Look for the most brilliantly colored vegetables, such as yellow squash, deep green spinach, sweet potatoes, and broccoli. Remember the darker the color, the more nutrients and antioxidants a vegetable contains.

The traditional DASH diet recommends four to five fruits a day, but if you are a woman and/or have a history of diabetes in your family, you might want to cut that back to two to three fruits a day. Fresh fruits are an irreplaceable source of nutrients like vitamin A, C, and vitamin E, and invaluable bioflavonoids. Perhaps the strongest link in pulmonary disease risk reduction and diet has been with solid fruits, and I urge you to include fruits at every meal. It's not difficult. For breakfast, you can toss in a tablespoon of raisins with your cereal; at lunch, you can have a piece of melon or apple; at night, you can enjoy a bowl of strawberries or a few slices of pineapple.

Low-fat or fat-free dairy products are very important on the DASH diet because they are sources of calcium and magnesium, which lower blood pressure. They are also excellent sources of protein and vitamin A. Remember that repeated epidemiological studies found that high vitamin A levels were linked to low pulmonary problem rates, and much of the source of vitamin A that we get is in dairy products. This does not just mean that you have to down two glasses of skim milk. You can use the milk in tea or coffee, you can have buttermilk, low-fat cheese, and/or fat-free yogurt (preferably unflavored or unsweetened).

Protein should be limited to about six ounces a day. That's two, three ounce servings, and that will probably be significantly less meat, chicken, or fish than most people are used to eating. The DASH diet cuts back on fat calories in protein and substitutes calories from grains, fruits, and vegetables, which contain vital nutrients. To keep cholesterol levels low, look for lean meats and cut away all visible fat, and broil or roast foods, rather than fry them.

The DASH diet is an evolving program and we are now looking at increasing levels of fish intake for hypertension and heart disease as well as for pulmonary problems. The American Heart Association recently revised its recommendations, and now includes eating one to two fish meals a week. I urge you to do that, since the omega-3 fatty acids in fish have also been linked to decreased levels of bronchial constriction.

In the laboratory, we have found that omega-3 fatty acids interrupt a body process known as the arachidonic acid cascade. When free radicals build up in the body, they lead to the production of chemicals that trigger the release of arachidonic acid, which in turn is converted to inflammatory mediators like the leukotrienes that cause bronchial constriction, leading to asthmatic attacks and wheezing. Omega-3 fatty acids block the production of arachidonic acid, stopping this unhealthy pattern before it has a chance to create problems. It is theorized that the lower levels of asthma in children and adults who have high fish intake may be linked to the effect of omega-3 fatty acids on arachidonic acid.

In the DASH diet, nuts and dry beans are also included several times a week. They are a wonderful source of energy, magnesium, potassium, fiber, and protein. Although they are too high in calories to be eaten every day, they are a good nutritional resource several times a week.

Fat intake is sharply limited in the DASH diet, and the recommendations are no more than a tablespoon of fat a day. This can include low-fat mayonnaise, salad oil, olive oil, and margarine. What type and how much fat is another area that's being explored in nutritional circles these days, and we are becoming increasingly interested in the benefits of olive oil in heart disease and cancer studies. There is some curiosity as to whether olive oil may have an anti-inflammatory and anti-irritating effect on the lungs, since Mediterranean countries have a high olive oil intake and a lower rate of lung disease. Using olive oil as your fat may turn out to be an additional benefit.

And finally, even sweets are permitted, albeit in very limited quantities, in the DASH diet. The idea that certain foods should be banned creates anxiety and pressures in my patients that lead to the complete failure of a diet. People begin to feel that if they sneak a little piece of chocolate or they use some jam on their toast that they've broken their diet and there's just no hope for them. Adding a little bit of sugar a few times a week will provide a sweetness and a pleasure in the diet that is necessary to stay with the program.

This is not a time-limited diet. You cannot reverse lung damage in eight weeks. You need to establish a healthy dietary pattern for you and your family to offer pulmonary protection and this needs to be a program you can live with.

The DASH diet offers additional benefits in my pulmonary patients, because pulmonary disease is often accompanied by cardiovascular problems. In many cases, the cigarette smoking

that led to the emphysema and chronic bronchitis has also affected heart function, and this low-cholesterol, blood-pressure-
lowering diet will be equally beneficial for a healthy heart. This
diet, which improves heart health, can only be beneficial for
the rest of the body.

One area where the DASH-II diet and I particularly agree is
in the sharp reduction of sodium. This is the only area where
some patients might feel that I'm taking something away from
them. But sodium appears to play a very important role in how
well and how easily we breathe. Sodium increases fluid volume
in the body, since the body tends to retain fluid, in order to
keep the concentration of sodium constant, and the more fluid
in the body, the harder the lungs and heart have to work to
function. By reducing sodium levels through diet, I can keep
the fluid volumes at a natural, healthy level. I have noticed in
my patients with chronic bronchitis and emphysema that when
I get them to reduce sodium intake, they find they often can
breathe better.

In the original DASH diet, doctors decided not to sharply
limit sodium because of the extra problems it causes in terms of
cooking and eating outside the home. Subsequently, low-
sodium versions of the DASH diet produced such dramatic improvement that sodium reductions are now part of the DASH
recommendations.

Interestingly, high-sodium diets have also been shown to be
linked to an increase in asthma risk and asthma symptoms. It
has been suggested that the sodium penetrates airway smooth
muscle cells altering calcium levels. This is felt to precipitate
bronchoconstriction. This does not mean that people with
asthma should avoid dairy products, since it's not the same kind

of calcium. This is an issue of the mechanics of the cellular sodium pump, and not dietary dairy products. I also believe that a low-sodium diet may also help prevent exacerbation attacks and the degree of symptoms in asthma.

Limiting salt intake is not as easy actually as limiting many other foods. Just taking the saltshaker off your table is a good first step, but it really will not adequately reduce your sodium intake. The average American consumes about six grams of sodium a day, and most diets recommend no more than two to three grams a day. In the newer DASH diets, they try to actually drop that level below the two-gram mark. Doctors find that people with high blood pressure do particularly well when they drop below the two-gram level.

It is important to recognize that most of the sodium that we eat is hidden in our foods. Some of it is there naturally. Dairy products and breads are very high in sodium. For example, a half a cup of cottage cheese can have 400 milligrams of sodium. Bread can have 200 milligrams per slice. Salt doesn't just provide flavor in baking, it also is involved in chemical reactions of dough formation and baking. It is actually very difficult for bakers to produce a soft flavorful bread without sodium.

Some other very common foods have incredibly high levels of sodium. Many condiments, such as ketchup, Worcestershire sauce, and mustard, are very high in sodium. Most canned soups have almost two grams a cup—more than your total daily intake on some DASH plans. Frozen foods, even diet frozen foods, have between half and one gram of sodium per serving. Sodium is put in because it makes the food taste better, it's an inexpensive seasoning, and it preserves food.

Limiting sodium, then, can be a challenge, and the best way

to avoid it is to buy foods as natural and fresh as possible. When eating in restaurants, request salads with olive oil and vinegar, rather than prepared dressing, and ask the waiter not to use salt when they broil or steam or poach your food.

A Lifetime Commitment

The DASH diet is not a short-term program; it is something to be followed for life. In order to follow anything for life, you need to be allowed a little freedom. I recommend that the majority of the time that you stay on the diet, but on special occasions, such as birthdays, holidays, and parties, you can relax certain restrictions on prepared foods in order not to lose enjoyment for the rest of your activities. But the next day you need to go right back onto your basic DASH program.

I find that it is possible to eat out practically everywhere on the DASH program. For example, in a Chinese restaurant, although most of the foods are very high in sodium, there is a wonderful variety of vegetables that are available to you. These nutrient-rich combos are perfect over brown rice.

In an Italian restaurant, you can always find green salads, grilled fish or veal or chicken, vegetables such as broccoli or spinach, and you can order a fresh fruit for dessert. In a Greek restaurant, there is a marvelous assortment of fresh vegetable salads, and this is the place to take advantage of bean salads, eggplant caviar, and tomato salads. You can find grilled lamb, grilled fish, steamed or sautéed Greek greens, and then there's usually melon for dessert. An Indian restaurant offers great vegetarian options. It's possible to get all five to seven servings of vegetables in one sitting, because there are so many wonderful vegetarian preparations, and those can be eaten with rice and baked, rather than fried, bread.

The restaurant food is going to be higher in sodium than food that you make yourself, but to compensate for the increased sodium, I would make sure that your restaurant choices are rich in the fresh fruits and vegetables and fish that seem to offer pulmonary protection in epidemiological studies. But you should not eat out like this every night, because you will be taking in more sodium than you want, which can both raise blood pressure as well as increase difficulty in breathing.

A Typical Day on the DASH Diet

A typical day on the DASH diet could start with a breakfast of cereal with some skim milk, raisins, and a sliced orange and tea or coffee. Lunch could be a tuna sandwich with lettuce, tomato, and onion, and an apple, and half a cup of yogurt. Dinner could be grilled chicken breasts with a baked sweet potato, broccoli, and a small dish of raspberries. This means you've got a bounty of brilliantly colored fruits and vegetables that offer nutrient value for the whole body, as well as following a dietary pattern that seems to reduce risk of pulmonary disease.

Weighty Matters

Weight, either too high or too low, can be part of pulmonary health problems. Excess body weight can make asthma control more difficult. For people with chronic bronchitis, studies have shown that as little as fifteen extra pounds above ideal weight can increase shortness of breath. I have found that the seden-

Following the DASH Diet

The DASH eating plan shown below is based on 2,000 calories a day. To lower the number of daily calories, limit yourself to the lower range of recommended servings for each of the food categories. The number of daily servings in a food group may vary from those listed depending on your caloric needs.

Use this chart to help you plan your menus or take it with you when you go to the store.

Food Groups	Grains	Vegetables	Fruits
Daily Servings	7–8	4–5	4–5
Serving Sizes	1 slice bread, 1 cup cereal,* ½ cup cooked rice, pasta, cereal	1 cup raw, ½ cup cooked, 6 oz. vegetable juice	6 oz. fruit juice, 1 medium fruit, ¼ cup dried fruit, ½ cup fresh or canned fruit
Examples	Whole wheat bread, English muffin, pita, bagel, cereals, grits, oatmeal	Tomatoes, lettuce, carrots, celery, squash, broccoli, spinach, green beans, peas, asparagus, zucchini, artichokes	Apples, berries, grapes, oranges, grapefruit, melons, mangoes, bananas, tangerines, cherries, plums, peaches
Health Benefits	Major sources of fiber, B vitamins	High in antioxidants, minerals, and fiber	Rich in vitamins, antioxidants, potassium

Dairy	Meats, fish, and poultry	Nuts, beans, and seeds	Fats and oils**	Sweets
2–3	2 or less	4–5 per week	2–3	5 per week
8 oz. milk, 1 cup yogurt, 1 oz. cheese	3 oz. cooked	2 tbsp. nuts or seeds, ½ cup cooked beans	1 tsp. margarine, 1 tbsp. low-fat mayonnaise, 2 tbsp. low-fat salad dressing, 1 tsp. vegetable oil	1 tbsp. jam, 1 tbsp. maple syrup, 8 oz. lemonade
Low-fat or fat-free milk; buttermilk; yogurt; cream, soy, or hard soy cheese	Lean beef, lamb, pork, chicken and turkey, salmon, tuna, eggs, shrimp, mussels, tofu	Almonds, walnuts, sunflower seeds, lentils, and kidney beans	Soft margarine, low-fat mayonnaise, low-fat salad dressing, olive oil	½ cup sorbet, jelly beans, jam, sugar, ices
Major sources of calcium and protein	Primary sources of protein and magnesium	Good source of minerals and healthy fats	Sources of essential fatty acids	Low-fat sweets add flavor to meals

*Serving sizes vary between ½–1¼ cups. Check products nutrition label.

**Fat content changes serving counts for fats and oils: For example, 1 tbsp. of regular salad dressing equals 1 serving; 1 tbsp. of a low-fat dressing equals ½ serving; 1 tbsp. of a fat-free dressing equals 0 servings.

tary habits of my patients play an important role in their weight gain. Higher activity levels that we recommend in exercise will not only increase the muscles in the body, it is also important for weight loss. The balance in a nutrient-rich diet will promote weight loss as it supplies optimum levels of nutrients.

When people become seriously ill and underweight, the DASH diet is a guide to the best possible food choices. Many of my patients with significant COPD are seriously undernourished. We find that eating leaves them breathless. As is common with many serious chronic problems, there may also be muscle loss and wasting, where the body seems to burn up calories at a faster rate.

We find that five to seven small meals are better tolerated than the traditional three meals a day schedule. It's not always possible to meet DASH goals, but it is a healthy standard at which to aim. Keep in mind that fiber can cause bloating, which is particularly unpleasant for people with COPD. To avoid the problem, try cooked, mashed, or puréed fruits and vegetables, in order to still take in the foods that offer pulmonary protection without unwanted side effects.

Chapter 7

The Pulmonary Protective Workout

D r. Schachter, have you been daydreaming?" my tiny but feisty patient demanded. "I just told you that making breakfast or washing my hair makes me short of breath. Now you want me to go out and exercise?" she admonished me in the same tone of voice she had probably used to terrify generations of students who were trying to explain to their history teacher why their homework was missing.

Struggling not to chuckle at being scolded like a schoolboy, I hastened to assure her I was not suggesting she buy a leotard and sign up for spin classes. Quite the contrary. Exercise can play a valuable role in pulmonary health, but it must be a specialized and well-monitored program.

This was not the first time that a patient had looked at me in disbelief when I brought up exercise. One of the reasons that I decided to write this book was to divert that look of panic when I start to introduce exercise options. Talking to patients over the years has shown me that it's important to explain how and why exercise will improve a wide range of health issues for them, not just pulmonary health, in order to give them confidence that an exercise program can be helpful.

For the past thirty years, scientists have accumulated an impressive body of evidence on the health benefits of exercise. For example, in a study of nearly 17,000 Harvard alumni, researchers found men who exercised several times a week had a 39 percent lower risk of heart attack. Exercise has an equally impressive record in hypertension. The same Harvard-based study found a 35 percent lower risk of high blood pressure in men who exercise regularly.

On the biochemical level, exercise has been shown to lower total blood cholesterol while raising the level of the "good" protective HDL cholesterol. Epidemiologists, who study patterns of cancer in different people, have found that exercise is associated with a lower risk of many cancers. For example, a study of 25,000 Norwegian women found that those who exercised at least four hours a week had a 37 percent lower risk of developing breast cancer. Similarly, a study of 1,000 women at the University of Southern California found that those who worked out 3.8 or more hours per week had only 50 percent the breast cancer rate of more sedentary women. Doctors believe that exercise decreases total estrogen output by your body. We also know that exercise is very important for weight control, as results from the National Weight Control Registry have demonstrated. A group of more than 1,000 men and women lost an average of sixty-four pounds over almost seven years. Follow-up visits showed that those study participants who exercised an hour or more a day were better able to keep the weight off than their less active colleagues. And finally, we have seen that exercise is important for emotional health. In a study done at the University of Virginia, 500 students were given a psychological profile. Results showed that 18 percent were clinically depressed. Some subjects were asked to jog three to five times a week, while others were told to refrain from exercise. After ten weeks, the emotional outlook of students who exercised was significantly improved. The sedentary group showed no changes.

A Healthy Heart and Lungs

There are actually three separate types of exercise—aerobics, weight training, and flexibility—and each of them plays an important role in pulmonary health.

Aerobic exercise builds cardiovascular fitness. A strong, slow, steady heartbeat is the foundation of a healthy body. A healthy cardiovascular system is essential for the delivery of oxygen to the cells, the ability of cells to use oxygen, and finally, for the blood vessels to carry away cellular waste products. Without adequate oxygen, every organ in the body suffers. Inadequate oxygen in the heart muscle leads to vascular disease and hypertension. In the brain, the result of a loss of oxygen is a decline in memory and an inability to reason. For the lungs, a lack of oxygen creates fatigue and shortness of breath.

To improve oxygen delivery, you need to build up cardiovascular fitness through regular aerobic exercise. The heart is a muscle that pumps blood throughout the body. As a muscle, it is made more efficient through aerobic exercise that gradually increases its ability to use oxygen more efficiently. Any exercise that increases heart rate, such as walking, biking, or swimming, increases the heart's ability to supply more oxygen with less effort. To build aerobic exercise, it is necessary to work the heart a minimum of twenty to thirty minutes a session, three times a week.

For many years, exercise physiologists and trainers believed that effective aerobic exercise had to be performed near or at the optimum training rate, a figure that is 60–80 percent of your maximum heart rate. This rate is estimated by your age subtracted from 220 beats per minute. For example, if you are fifty years old, your estimated maximum heart rate for aerobic exercise is 170, and 80 percent of 170 is 136; your minimum heart rate would be 60 percent or 102. Consequently, your exercise heart rate should be between 102 and 136. To keep track of your heart rate, we suggested that you take your pulse for ten seconds while exercising, then multiply that by six to get the heart rate per minute.

This is a lot of monitoring and calculation to do while jogging on a treadmill and impossible to do while swimming or biking. Physicians felt that lesser levels of exercise would not increase fitness. We were wrong. This type of no-pain, no-gain approach to exercise is neither possible nor necessary for people with pulmonary problems. We now know that lower levels of exercise work to improve fitness. In other words, exercise does not have to be punishing to provide important physical benefits.

During aerobic exercise, the body needs additional amounts of oxygen. The heart needs to pump more blood with each beat and with exercise it becomes more efficient. Doing this type of exercise allows muscle arteries to dilate so that more blood can be carried to the muscles. This makes it easier for the heart to move blood throughout the body, a change which also lowers blood pressure numbers. The increased blood flow influences new capillary formation and encourages collateral circulation that helps to increase blood supply to the muscles.

All of these factors assist the heart, allowing it to work better with less effort. For the lungs, the most important benefits of aerobic exercise is that the muscles throughout the body become more efficient at absorbing oxygen from the blood. This means the lungs do not have to work as hard to supply oxygen. If the lungs are damaged, they eventually can no longer provide the oxygen the body needs, resulting in fatigue and shortness of breath. With exercise, muscles can become more efficient and now obtain more oxygen because of improved circulation. Increased oxygen levels provide more energy and relieve feelings of fatigue.

Weight Training

Weight training for pulmonary patients does not mean training to compete for Mister or Miss Universe. Gentle, well-monitored, resistance workouts, either with elastic bands or light weights, can improve pulmonary function. As your muscles work against weights, or a resistance, microscopic tears develop in the fibers and they split. As they heal, new muscle mass is formed and the size of the muscle is increased. This larger muscle is more efficient.

Over time, this increase in muscle mass increases the work capacity of the muscle. For the pulmonary system, the increase in muscle volume and efficiency leads to a greater capacity to absorb oxygen from the blood. As a result, there is better oxygenation of the body without an increased demand on the lungs. In other words, you will feel less fatigue and shortness of breath for the same level of work.

Flexibility

The ability of the body to move joints and ligaments through their full range of motion is known as flexibility. Bending over to touch your toes is a popular and simple way to judge lower body flexibility. For the upper body, wrap your right hand behind your right shoulder, then reach up behind your back with your left hand and try to grasp the fingers of the right hand. This is a much harder test than toe touching, but upper body flexibility is critical for optimum pulmonary function.

When lungs have to struggle to work properly, we start to use the muscles in our chest, neck, and shoulders to help the lungs function. This tends to tighten up the upper body and robs strength from the other functions of these large muscles. This can be felt when you raise your hands to hang curtains, or use a hair dryer. This is why my patient became breathless when she washed her hair. If you begin to feel short of breath, it is because the shoulder muscles needed for these tasks are already working hard to help your lungs. We are going to suggest flexibility exercises to uncramp the muscles while employing weights to increase their strength.

Establishing Fitness Levels

If you've ever picked up a book on exercise, you have probably read the suggestion to see a doctor before you do an exercise program. This is especially critical and necessary for people with pulmonary problems. We need to develop an extensive cardiopulmonary profile to be able to devise a safe and effective program for each person. Traditional programs will tell you to see a doctor if you are over forty, or have a heart condition. Perhaps the doctor will listen to your heart and occasionally do a stress test. When pulmonary problems are an issue, you will need to do an extensive workup that is available in cardiopulmonary labs and this is, in most cases, covered by private insurance, HMOs, and Medicare.

Cardiac stress testing is routinely recommended before beginning an exercise program if there are underlying health problems or you are over age forty-five. By running on a treadmill while hooked up to an electrocardiogram (EKG), we can assess heart rate, pick up irregular rhythm and signs of coronary blockage.

For people with COPD, we need an enhanced stress test that measures how the respiratory system can function under the increased work demands of exercise.

In addition to the EKG, we include three tests: you will breathe through a mouthpiece connected to a spirometer and special gas monitors to measure levels of O_2 and CO_2, as well as the volume of air that passes in and out of the lungs. To gauge blood pressure, we'll attach a blood pressure cuff to your arm. Finally, we'll attach a pulse oximeter painlessly to your finger to measure oxygen saturation as you exercise.

The pulse oximeter shines a light onto the skin which measures the amount of O_2 bound to hemoglobin. In people without heart or pulmonary problems, the O_2 saturation ranges between 95 and 100 percent. When O_2 saturation drops below 90 percent the heart is placed under excessive strain. If O_2 saturation becomes too low during exercise, we supply extra O_2

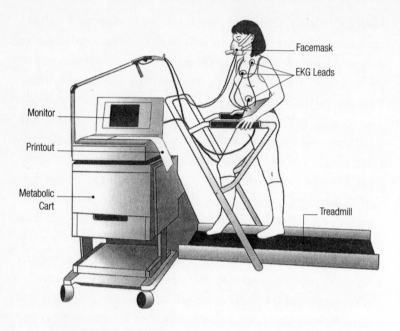

Cardiopulmonary stress testing allows a physician to judge how well
your heart and lungs respond to different levels of exercise. If the
oxygen level of your blood drops too low, we know that supplemental
oxygen will help you get the benefits of an exercise program.

to help you exercise safely. We can feed additional oxygen
through a nasal tube that draws it from a tank.

Once we have an idea of your pulmonary and cardiac status,
we can develop a program to meet your needs. There are actually three different types of exercise programs. One for asthmatics, another for people who are diagnosed with COPD, and
the third for either current or former smokers who are not
symptomatic but are certainly at increased risk for developing
pulmonary problems.

The carefully monitored exercise program for people with

COPD is done in an eight-to-ten-week session in a pulmonary rehabilitation center. Fortunately, it is usually covered by Medicare, private insurance, and HMOs. Usually, there is one physical therapist who works with four to six patients at a time. The goals of the program are very different from those you'll find at Gold's Gym. We are not trying to train for a triathlon. The goals are to build muscle to improve oxygen delivery to reduce risk of cardiac disease, and to increase stamina.

Studies have shown that these programs can provide measurable benefits. For example, researchers at the University of Connecticut School of Medicine reported that just twelve exercise sessions over a six-week period produced a measurable increase in fitness. Training included using a treadmill, a StairMaster, a stationary bike, and rubber stretching strips called Therabands, for flexibility and strength training. Each session gradually increased the workload of the previous day. At the end of six weeks, there was, on the average, a 30 percent increase in exercise capacity as measured by the distance walked in twelve minutes. Even more encouraging was the fact that the people with the lowest fitness levels at the start of the program showed the greatest degree of improvement. In other words, it is never too late to get in shape.

The aerobic component of the exercise is done on a stationary bike or a treadmill. When you start doing exercise, you are carefully monitored for both pulmonary and cardiac changes so that we can track your heart rate and, most importantly, we can follow the oxygenation of your blood. People with COPD tend to desaturate, or experience a drop in blood levels of oxygen from the stress of exercise. We certainly don't want you to go too low. That will lead to breathlessness and perhaps a sense of suffocation and panic. The monitor is placed on your finger and will measure your oxygen saturation.

From your exercise testing, we will have a good idea of how much and how quickly you can perform exercise. If you feel breathless, we will often supply oxygen while you are exercising, in order for you to be able to work out for extended periods of time on a stationary bike or treadmill. If leg muscles are particularly weak, we start off with the stationary bike, which will quickly improve the lower body strength. We can either use it singly, or in combination with the treadmill, depending on what form of exercise you like better, or what exercise is better for your physical needs.

The arm bike will exercise the muscles of your upper body. You simply sit in a chair and rotate a winch and your arms will move much like your legs would on a bicycle. This is a very helpful workout for those upper body muscles that are so important for assisting breathing.

To build up muscle strength, we have you use very light weights (1–2 lbs.) in a series of exercises to put resistance on muscles. I find they are very good for people who haven't exercised in a while because we can start with a relatively small resistance and not exhaust deconditioned muscles.

Flexibility exercises can be particularly important for the upper body. We want to loosen up those cramped accessory muscles that have become involved in assisted breathing. We can do three or four upper body exercises to stretch out the body. For example, a Theraband exercise starts by standing on the elastic band and pulling it until there is tension. Adjust the tension in the bands and raise your arms to shoulder height. Still at shoulder height, swing your arms out to your side and back to the center. Repeat each exercise several times.

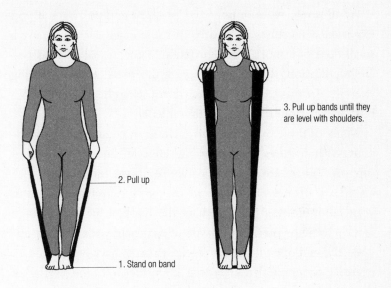

2. Pull up

3. Pull up bands until they are level with shoulders.

1. Stand on band

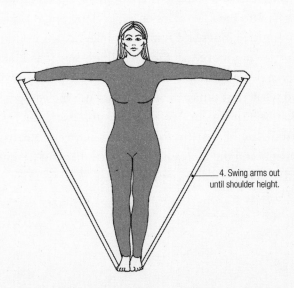

4. Swing arms out until shoulder height.

Using elasticized rubber bands known as Therabands can improve upper body strength and flexibility.

At all times, we monitor your progress and pull back if you experience shortness of breath. In some cases, we might use a small dose of a short acting bronchodilator. Usually called rescue medication, we use it to prevent shortness of breath during exercise. In this case, you start off the exercise session with a puff or two from the short-acting inhaler.

Many of these programs also include an educational component with lectures on nutrition, lifestyle, and psychological support. They are an invaluable resource for people with COPD. I strongly recommend that you search them out in your community. At the back of the book, I have a resource section to help you find this type of facility in your community.

At the end of eight to ten weeks, patients have established an exercise program that they can continue at home. Many of them continue and expand the program by incorporating a daily walk into their activities or by working out at a traditional gym, using treadmills and stationary bikes. Keep in mind, you will not be monitored at these facilities, but it is hoped that after three to four months in a structured facility, you will have learned what your limits are and how to use the equipment in a way that best suits your needs. If you stop exercising, you will retain some of the benefits for a while but, over time, these improvements and the increased endurance that you have worked so hard to acquire will disappear.

In a small study done in Glasgow, doctors found that electrical stimulation of leg muscles can improve whole body strength and breathing ability. Muscle stimulation was applied to thigh muscles fifteen minutes a day, five times a week. At the end of six weeks, doctors reported that patients had better oxygen uptake and more energy. Further tests are under way to learn if electrical muscle stimulation should be recommended as a standard feature of pulmonary rehabilitation.

Exercising with Asthma

Most asthmatics experience a tightness or a wheezing upon exertion, and anyone with a long history of asthma tends to know that running and physical exertion can trigger an asthma attack. In fact, between 80 to 100 percent of asthmatics will experience symptoms upon exercise, but this does not mean asthmatics cannot exercise. The list of elite and Olympic athletes that have asthma is impressive, including Jackie Joyner Kersey, Dennis Rodman, Greg Louganis, and Aaron Carver. In fact, up to 40 percent of elite athletes in different sports experience a type of exercise-induced bronchospasm, or asthma, at high levels of exertion.

I have found that many asthmatic patients, because they experience discomfort from asthma, shrink away from physical activity. This is unfortunate because it creates a cycle that actually decreases general health. If people with asthma find that they become breathless from exercise, then they become more sedentary. The more sedentary they become, the more their muscles weaken. They are less able to transport oxygen around, which increases breathing problems.

Exercise is an extremely important component for asthma control and I encourage all my asthmatics to stay active. But, like my patients with COPD, asthmatics need to be fully evaluated before beginning a program. Most exercise books and experts will advise people who are over forty, or who have heart conditions, to seek medical evaluation before beginning an exercise program. With asthma, whatever your age, and whatever your physical condition, you need to have exercise stress testing for cardiopulmonary evaluation before beginning any exercise program.

When Exercise Makes Asthma Worse

Sitting on a gurney in the emergency room, Bruce Taggert looked very worried. Recently divorced at thirty-five, he had decided to get in shape and lose those twenty pounds that he had gained since college. He bought a pair of the latest ergonomically correct running shoes and set out to run off the weight. He felt pretty good for the first ten minutes, then his chest became tight and he found it difficult to breathe. By the time Bruce saw his doctor, he felt fine, and the EKG showed no abnormalities. But when he tried running again, the symptoms recurred. This time he went straight to an emergency room, where another EKG was normal. Because he was also complaining of a cough, I was called in to take a look.

Talking to Bruce, I learned that he had seasonal allergies to ragweed and his mother had asthma. Further pulmonary function tests confirmed my suspicions—Bruce had exercise-induced asthma, or EIA.

Exercise-induced asthma results from a narrowing of the

airways following exertion. About 90 percent of people with asthma experience the symptoms to some degree. For people like Bruce, it can be the first time they realize that an asthma problem exists. Fortunately, EIA is one of the most preventable and/or treatable forms of asthma. In fact, many competitive athletes with EIA continue to break records and win medals. Interestingly, about 10 percent of people without asthma will develop similar symptoms after exercise.

Causes of Exercise-Induced Asthma

While doctors do not fully understand the precise mechanisms behind EIA, we have identified a number of key factors. We realize the temperature of the air we breathe is important to airway control. Under resting situations, most of the air we breathe is inhaled through the nose, where it is moistened by body fluids and warmed to body temperature before reaching the lungs. During exercise, we tend to breathe through the mouth. As a result, the air is dry and cool when it reaches the airways, leading to bronchial irritability and constriction. This effect is particularly rapid when you exercise in colder weather. Ice skating, skiing, and running in winter can precipitate asthma symptoms.

To make matters worse, when we breathe through our mouths, we gulp in large amounts of pollutants that are suspended in the air. We believe that this increased level of environmental irritants may also set off hyperactive airways.

Fortunately, exercise-induced asthma responds well to a range of strategies. Simply wrapping a scarf over your nose and mouth in cold, dry weather may be all you need to avoid EIA.

In the summer months, a small face mask will serve the same purpose. Changing the type of sport will often be all that is needed. The warm humid conditions of swimming are far less likely to cause EIA than running or cycling. Exercising indoors in a climate-controlled gym will also limit exposure to pollen, pollution, and cold dry air.

Many of my patients with irritable airways use their short-acting beta-agonist inhaler before beginning exercise or sports. Normally, we call these rescue medications, but when used with EIA, we call them preventive therapy. A quick puff before exercise will stabilize the mast cells, preventing their release of bronchoconstricting compounds.

The Asthma-Friendly Exercise Program

If you have tried to exercise but have been unable to stick with it, there are also eight-to-ten-week programs to create pulmonary fitness for asthmatics, and I urge you to find them in your community. Similar to the programs for patients with chronic obstructive lung disease, they have been shown to not only improve fitness but also to decrease symptoms and, in some cases, reduce medication needs. For example, a study from Sweden found that a ten-week structured exercise program dramatically improved health and fitness in asthmatics. The training was carried out in a warm swimming pool. All the participants were led through a vigorous forty-five-minute interval program five days a week for two weeks, then twice a week for eight more weeks. At the end of the study researchers found a 25 percent increase in forced vital capacity, representing a significant improvement in pulmonary function. Even more encouraging was the fact that during the training period, the number of emergency room visits for asthmatic attacks dropped more than 60 percent.

Swimming Pool Asthma

For many patients, swimming is a wonderful exercise. It provides a great aerobic workout without a strain on the joints. In theory, the warm moist air could be a healthy environment for people with sensitive lungs. Unfortunately, fumes from the chlorine added to most pools can be irritating to already hyperactive airways. In fact, researchers from the University of Birmingham in England found that many lifeguard and swimming teachers actually developed occupational asthma from their jobs. Moreover, a highly publicized study in Belgium found that school-age children who swam regularly in highly chlorinated pools had early signs of lung injury. To avoid pulmonary hazards, I prefer that my patients swim in an ocean or a lake whenever possible.

Warming up and cooling down before an exercise also seems to prevent asthma bronchospasm. We suspect that it allows the airways to adjust gradually to the new demands that the exercise places upon them.

I find that for the weight training component of an asthma exercise program, two-to-five-pound free weights can be used very successfully to increase upper body strength. Like people with chronic bronchitis or emphysema, asthmatics can use the increased muscle strength to provide increased oxygenation to the body.

Most younger asthmatics have the strength to be able to use free weights very successfully. These can be done either at home, or in a gym.

Weight training can be done with two- to five-pound free weights for upper body strength. For lower body strength, you can use traditional floor and leg exercises, such as lunges and squats. Never work out above your capacity, and if you feel yourself developing tightness in your chest, stop exercising that day.

An additional benefit for asthmatics is that the increased exercise will almost invariably result in a weight loss, which is very beneficial for most asthmatics. The less weight you're carrying means that your heart and lungs have less body mass to supply oxygen to; this will usually translate to a lessening of symptoms. A study published in the *British Medical Journal* reported that overweight asthmatic women showed improvement when they lost weight. After a fourteen-week weight loss program, participants had improved lung function, less shortness of breath, and less need of medication.

For smokers or former smokers who do not have any pulmonary symptoms but are still concerned about their pulmonary health, I suggest a cardiopulmonary stress testing to see if there are subclinical changes in your pulmonary and cardiac functions. If you have no sign of problems, you may have not yet reached the critical number of pack years as a smoker. You are probably under forty or are just born with lucky genetic programming to be able to resist the damages of smoking. This doesn't mean that you should continue smoking, but it does indicate that you can undertake an exercise program without supervision.

Now is the time to start a traditional and dedicated exercise program to improve the fitness of your entire body. Remember that smoking not only affects your lungs but your heart as well. The impact of having smoked on the heart can be offset by a full-fledged aerobic and strength-training program. You should start a progressive exercise program that starts slowly and builds in challenge and intensity. Start with a walking program, where you walk briskly for twenty to thirty minutes, then work up to an hour. When you can walk a mile in twelve minutes, graduate to running.

If you start to experience problems, such as breathlessness, a sense of constriction, or coughing, especially when you exercise outdoors, you may have early lung damage that we are just not picking up at this point. In this situation, I would switch workouts to be indoors on a stationary bike or on a treadmill. Again, never exceed your comfort zone. Do not let yourself be bullied into working to the traditional 65 to 85 percent of maximum heart rate. This is an intensive level of exercise, and you need to work up to this level. People who are smokers, or even former smokers, need to work up to such levels even more gradually, and may never be able to exercise at that intensity.

Getting Hard

Muscle strength is characterized by the ability to lift a relatively heavy weight for a short period of time, while endurance is the ability to lift a light weight repeatedly and quickly over a longer period of time. Strength and endurance are clearly related, and both employ weight training to condition muscles. You can build up strength very quickly, using isokinetic exercises with weight machines. Weights usually start at ten pounds and can go all the way up to hundreds of pounds. You should work with a trainer who will focus on both strength training and endurance.

Strength is developed through progressive training. Weights are applied to normal body movements, such as bending the elbow or the knee. The weight overloads the muscle, forcing it to contract at maximum capacity. Gains are made most quickly from heavy resistance and few repetitions, then the muscles are allowed to recuperate for at least twenty-four hours until the next training session. Each session calls for four to eight repetitions, which is equal to one set for each muscle group.

Endurance can be developed in a program of curl-ups and push-ups. The repetition is key, gradually increasing the number that can be done before exhaustion. For example, when you first start out, you may be able to complete just five curl-ups. Over the next month, you will gradually be able to increase this to fifteen curl-ups, with the same effort you took to complete the first.

Weight training machines offer distinct benefits over free weights. They have heavier weights and can work through the full range of motion more smoothly, improving and strengthening the length of the entire muscle. Isokinetic machines also isolate muscles precisely so that you can know exactly what muscles you are working on. I have found them to be very safe, yet effective. You can't drop them on your foot, or overextend yourself on the muscles. If it is too heavy, you just let go.

You particularly want to work on the large muscle groups in the lower body, the legs and the upper body, the arms and shoulders. These are the large muscles that your lungs are going to struggle with to deliver oxygen.

Lie on the floor, arms folded, knees bent, feet on the floor.

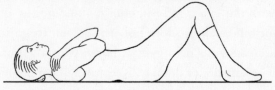

Pull up slowly into a sitting position.

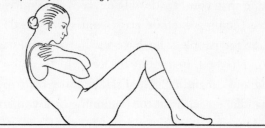

Curl body into knees, hold for 3 seconds, then roll back to floor.

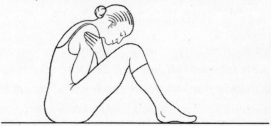

Curl-ups can increase the strength of your back and abdomen.

Using the machines, you will use the weight of the machines to provide resistance to build strength. For the endurance exercises, you will use the weight of your own body to provide the resistance to your muscles. In a traditional workout program, you will alternate days between aerobic activities, such as walking or treadmill and stationary bike workout, with days where you do weight training. If you don't need monitoring, you can either work out in a gym or in your own home.

If your schedule just does not permit you to go to a gym, you can create your own gym at home with a stationary bike and a set of barbells, or dumbbells that weigh ten pounds. Using just a few pieces of equipment, you can create a first-rate workout routine that you can do whenever it fits your schedule. I don't advise joining exercise classes unless they're designed for smokers or for people who have cardio or pulmonary health problems. They can be too fast-paced, which can be both discouraging and exhausting. They can be more than you're really able to handle, especially at the beginning or if you continue to smoke.

Stretching Toward Health

Flexibility exercises are equally important, to keep stretching out the new muscles that you are developing, and to prevent injury from your aerobic running or exercise programs. Swimming is also an excellent option for the aerobic program, if you have access to a pool.

Before beginning a flexibility program, you should start by measuring just how flexible you are. Take this test to find out:

Flexibility Test

- Tape a line on the floor as shown on page 154.
- Place a yardstick so that the line is even with the 15" mark
- Sit on the floor so your heels are on the line and about 5" apart
- With legs straight, bend forward as far as you can and touch the stick.
- Compare your stretch to the box below

Men	Ages 36–45	Age 46+
Excellent	20	19
Good	14–19	13–18
Fair	6–13	6–12
Poor	<5	5 or less

Women	Ages 36–45	Age 46+
Excellent	22	21
Good	17–21	16–20
Fair	11–16	10–15
Poor	10 or less	9 or less

Flexibility helps you to enjoy your aerobic and weight training workouts. It allows you to get the full advantage of the extension of muscles and the building of strength.

For former smokers without symptoms, these fitness programs benefit overall cardiopulmonary health. Exercise cannot overcome the impact of the damage done by smoking, but it can strengthen your body. We do not know if this can prevent chronic obstructive lung disease, but we have seen that by increasing muscle strength and increasing the capacity to provide oxygen to the body, you can relieve or delay symptoms of breathlessness and fatigue that are characteristic of chronic obstructive lung disease. It is important that you start your exercise program now, whatever your age, for pulmonary health.

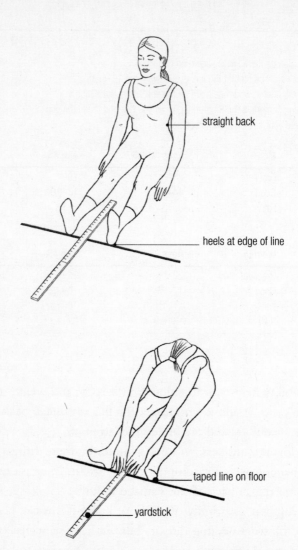

straight back

heels at edge of line

taped line on floor

yardstick

Judging how far you can reach over the line will give you an idea of
your current flexibility and a way to judge the progress
of your exercise program.

Chapter 8

It's Never Too Late to Quit

Chuck Matusik looked and talked like the labor lawyer he was. A longtime smoker, he had chronic obstructive bronchitis that left him breathless. He came to me after he quit smoking because his continuing shortness of breath made it difficult for him to deliver his usual winning arguments in court. He did well on the medications I prescribed and came back a few times in the year that followed. Then he stopped coming into my office, but called regularly for prescription refills or requests for antibiotics to treat repeated episodes of respiratory infections. Finally, I told him I needed to see him before I could renew his medications. When he came in, he confessed sheepishly that he had stayed away because he was embarrassed. He had started to smoke again.

I quickly assured Chuck that I would never judge him. Cigarettes are as addictive as alcohol or cocaine, and relapse is a reflection of their powerfully addictive qualities and not a personal reflection on him. People do not smoke because they are weak-willed, stupid, lazy, or self-destructive. They smoke because nicotine addiction can be even harder to overcome than addiction to illicit drugs. In this chapter, I will explore how nicotine affects your body and your mind and offer the successful combination smoking cessation program that provides both psychological and physical support.

Quick Tip

If you have started smoking again, please don't avoid seeing your doctor. He will not judge you, but you need to get medical attention for your ongoing pulmonary problem. If he makes you feel uncomfortable, get another doctor.

The Bright, Golden Leaf of Disaster

The tobacco plant is native to the United States, and Native Americans were using tobacco products in the Americas well before the time of Columbus. Throughout the eighteenth and nineteenth centuries, tobacco was consumed in chewing tobacco, snuff, pipes, and cigars.

Cigarette smoking as a habit didn't really start until the early part of the twentieth century. Prior to 1884, a good cigarette roller could produce just 2,000 cigarettes a day. The mechanized rollers at the turn of the century could roll out 120,000 cigarettes daily. In 1892, the invention of safety matches allowed smokers to carry around a quick and easy means for lighting up, turning cigarettes into a source of instant gratification.

The cigarette habit as we have come to know it today really became prevalent in the United States during the Second World War. During the 1940s, cigarette companies distributed free cigarettes to our soldiers abroad and essentially hooked a whole generation on the cigarette habit.

There were clues as early as the 1930s that cigarette smoking could cause health problems. Most of the observations came from Europe, and they did not make a big impact in the United States, but in 1950, a study published in the *Journal of the American Medical Association* for the first time linked cigarette smoking to lung cancer. It showed that smokers had up to a thirteen-fold increased risk of lung cancer. The results sparked an unprecedented effort to help explain the effects of tobacco on health.

President Kennedy designed a council to review the evidence, and in 1964 the report from the Surgeon General was the first in a series of documents that summarized the knowledge about smoking and health. There have since been twenty-one reports from the Surgeon General's office linking smoking to specific diseases, examining nicotine addiction, and outlining the benefits of smoking cessation. As Antonio Novella, Surgeon General in 1990, said, "It is safe to say that smoking represents the most extensively documented cause of disease ever investigated in the history of biomedical research."

The Downside of Equality

The pattern of smoking among women was originally quite different from that of men. In the early 1900s, when cigarette smoking first became prevalent, men started to smoke in their teenage years, while women took on the habit at a much later age. It has only been more recently, with changes in our society that go along with equal rights for women, that cigarette companies have seen an opportunity to market cigarettes for women in the same way they market them for men. Now the pattern of starting to smoke in women is the same of that in men. In other words, women like men begin smoking as teenagers and they're addicted to it by the time they're in their twenties. We can see the results of this smoking pattern in the recent health statistics that show there has been a sharp rise in heart disease, lung cancer, and COPD rates among women— the latter a 100 percent rise in the past decade.

A Nation of Reluctant Smokers

If you ask them, most people who smoke want to quit. Given what is known about the health effects of smoking, and the current climate of social disapproval, nine out of ten adult smokers wish they could wake up tomorrow morning as non-smokers.

Smoking Is a Family Affair

A single cigarette smoker in a family is a tremendous incentive for everyone else to smoke. Committed smokers buy cigarettes by the carton and it is very easy for teenagers to slip out a few cigarettes or even a whole pack without the parents' knowledge. If you eliminate adult smokers in the home, then the habit has to begin outside the family. Young people have to buy and pay for their own cigarettes, and are forced to smoke on the sly. It is certainly not an impossible situation, and many teenagers do try to smoke at least for some time, but the social and the family context plays a large role in cigarette addiction.

It's No Longer Cool to Smoke

The move to help people quit smoking is part of a general increased consciousness in health. People exercise more, watch their diet, know their cholesterol numbers, and are aware that cigarettes are just bad for you. Life and health insurance plans can cost more for smokers. New legislation has limited the number of places that people can smoke. Nationwide, smoking has been banned in office buildings, buses, subways, taxis, planes, hospitals, and schools. In many states, smoking is banned or restricted in restaurants. Public awareness campaigns from the American Cancer Society, the National Institutes of Health, and the American Lung Association have made people uncomfortably aware of the health hazards associated with smoking. They point out that one in five deaths in America are associated with cigarettes. Even more troubling, 40,000 people die unnecessarily each year as the result of simply living or working with people who smoke. The 4,000 toxins in the smoke cause heart disease, lung cancer, and pulmonary problems in nonsmokers who are exposed to cigarettes.

The impact of these public education campaigns has been significant. Smoking rates are down for both men and women. Less than 25 percent of adult Americans now smoke, whereas in the 1950s, more than half of all adults were smokers. Forty million Americans can rightfully consider themselves ex-smokers. Unfortunately, there are still 50 million Americans hooked on nicotine and it is estimated that each day another 3,000 teenagers start smoking.

Why Is It So Hard to Quit?

It's become clear to doctors that an addiction to cigarettes is as strong an addiction as that to heroin and cocaine. We know this because the success rate for people trying to quit heroin, cocaine, and cigarettes is almost identical.

With cigarettes, the addictive compound is nicotine, and the modern cigarette can best be described as a nicotine delivery system. When you inhale the smoke of a cigarette, all the by-products formed by the burning cigarette are drawn into the lungs and enter the bloodstream through the alveoli. The effect is as if you had taken a solution of nicotine, filled it up in a syringe, and injected it into your veins.

Nicotine is an amine, a type of compound that has a broad number of physiological effects. For example, it acts not only in the brain, where it causes addiction, but on the smooth muscle of the blood vessels, where it raises blood pressure. Nicotine also affects the smooth muscle of the GI tract, increasing digestion—which is probably why people who smoke like to light up after meals. For many years, doctors actually recommended cigarettes for gastrointestinal disorders, such as chronic irritable bowel syndrome.

Nicotine can both stimulate and relax you. In small doses, when you take small quick puffs, it is stimulating. You feel sharper, more alert, and studies have actually shown that nicotine enhances attention span and memory. In large doses, when you inhale deeply with long draws on the cigarette, the nicotine has a calming effect and reduces feelings of stress.

The manufacturing process of tobacco can influence the amount of nicotine in individual cigarettes. In the United

States, most cigarettes are made with blonde tobacco, which is dried under specific conditions known as curing. In Europe and outside the United States, cigarettes are made with dark tobacco with higher nicotine levels.

How Nicotine Creates Cravings

One of the effects of nicotine and the one that is felt to be associated with addiction is the resetting of the chemical responses in parts of the brain that secrete dopamine. This chemical is not necessarily associated with pleasure, but with the *anticipation* of pleasure. Once the cells that secrete dopamine have been reset by nicotine (or by cocaine or heroin), it takes larger and larger doses of the drug to keep that center stimulated and the levels of dopamine to be maintained. In the absence of the drug, what the person experiences is not the absence of pleasure, but the absence of the anticipation of pleasure. In other words, you become apathetic and depressed. This is the rationale behind some of the newest therapies for nicotine addiction, which involve the use of antidepressant medications, to act specifically on these dopamine centers.

The anxiety and depression withdrawal symptoms are linked to the absence of the anticipation of pleasure. This lengthy withdrawal from nicotine forms the basis for another strategy, using nicotine replacement with a patch or gum.

The Psychology of Smoking

Like alcohol and heroin, we become addicted to cigarettes in a social context, and the drug becomes part of that context. To withdraw from the drug implies not only physical withdrawal but also a withdrawal that accompanies a breaking of these emotional and social ties. If you are addicted to heroin, getting off the drug means you have to structure your life differently. The same is true for cigarette smoking. It can be as simple as the fact that you anticipate lighting up a cigarette during certain activities, such as after eating, taking a drink, having a cup of coffee, or during times of stress. All of these situations which people associate with "beneficial effects" of cigarette smoking make it all the harder to quit the habit.

In addition, we are very orally oriented animals, and cigarette smoking gives us something to do with our mouth and our hands. For many people, this is an important part of the addiction in social situations. Where normally they have something to keep them busy, they are now left to their own devices.

The Psychology of Quitting

Most people who try to quit do so on their own. They don't go to meetings, take medication, or use patches. They do it by going cold turkey because their motivation is so high. My mother-in-law Martha had smoked at least a pack a day since she was fifteen years old. Not even a bad pneumonia that left her weak and breathless for months stopped her smoking habit. One day when she went to a doctor for a routine visit, she sat in the waiting room with a man who was struggling to breathe, even though he was using a portable oxygen tank. When she saw him unhook the oxygen to light up a cigarette, she decided on the spot to quit and she never smoked another cigarette.

Unfortunately, for the majority of people who attempt to

quit cold turkey, this strategy is not successful. Results show that only about 10 percent of people can quit without assistance. But trying to do it on your own should never be discouraged. People develop their own methods that work for them, and everyone's approach is different. They may try to wean themselves off smoking, limiting themselves to a specific number of cigarettes each day. It has been my experience that abstaining completely works better than trying to quit gradually. Going cold turkey does make sense. People who try to reduce the number of cigarettes to a point where they feel uncomfortable find it very easy to slip back into their old habits. Anybody who smokes at least five to ten cigarettes a day is still considered addicted.

I never want to discourage anybody from trying to quit, whatever their approach. The important thing about smoking cessation is making up your mind that you want to try. Statistically, each time you attempt to quit, you have a one in ten chance of succeeding. The more times you try, the greater the overall odds are that you will be successful.

Not infrequently, I will have a patient who has had a life-altering situation that enables them to quit. They either have a heart attack, develop pneumonia, become pregnant, or are hospitalized for respiratory failure and have to be on a ventilator. Then, of course, they can't smoke and, as a result, they have ten to twenty days without cigarettes. When they are released from the hospital, they find they can indeed live without smoking. If they are lucky, they won't relapse and they stay ex-smokers. Unfortunately, it seems to take a major catastrophe for these cases to succeed, and I'd love for you to avoid this doomsday approach to smoking cessation.

Beating the Odds

Despite the very best motivation and commitment, 90 percent of people who try fail to kick the habit. To improve these odds, doctors analyzed quitting behaviors and have come up with six stages for quitting:

Stage 1: Pre-contemplation

The smoker has no desire to quit. They like to smoke and as one of my patients put it "quitting is off the table."

Stage 2: Contemplation

The smoker starts to think about quitting. They are not yet at the point where they look into different ways to help themselves quit, but the idea is always at the back of their mind. Sometimes they even raise the issue with their physician, expressing concern about the impact of smoking on their health. I've learned not to force the issue at this point. Not infrequently, people stall at this level, becoming what we call "chronic contemplators." They worry about their smoking habits, but don't take additional steps.

Stage 3: Preparation

The smoker starts to take concrete steps. They may buy a book or tape on quitting, switch to low-tar cigarettes, or cut back on the number they light up.

Stage 4: Action

The smoker actually stops smoking. They are anxious yet proud of their smoke-free status.

Stage 5: Maintenance

Now off cigarettes for at least six months, the smoker feels confident that tobacco is no longer part of their lives.

Stage 6: Relapse

Whether a result of increased stress or the reassertion of old habits, the smoker begins to use cigarettes again. Former ex-smokers like my patient Chuck Matusik are embarrassed by their "failure" and frightened that they will never be able to quit. It is important that you understand that relapse is part of the normal recovery process. Learning what cues the use of cigarettes for you will help you succeed the next time you try to quit.

The Support You Need

When I began to practice pulmonary medicine, all we could offer smokers was sympathy. It was painful to see smart, motivated patients unable to quit the habit that was destroying their health. With the introduction of nicotine replacement, I was finally able to provide concrete assistance and the success rate for smoking cessation increased two- to three-fold.

The idea of nicotine replacement therapy is a very simple one. Nicotine is the addictive agent in cigarettes, and it is the sudden withdrawal from this drug that causes physical and emotional distress symptoms. In order to prevent these often severe withdrawal symptoms, we use a replacement strategy. Instead of the nicotine in the cigarettes, you receive it from another delivery system that doesn't affect the lungs. Smoking activates large numbers of nicotine receptors in the brain.

When these receptors get their fix of nicotine, it improves your mood, curbs your appetite, and relieves tension. When you quit smoking, the receptors don't get their required nicotine, causing you to feel depressed and anxious. Nicotine replacement therapy does not provide the same sensation as a cigarette, but it supplies enough nicotine to block withdrawal symptoms.

The nicotine patches are formulated in different strengths and are available without a prescription. The patches have an adhesive backing that sticks naturally to the skin. A fresh patch is used every day to deliver twenty-four hours of nicotine to the bloodstream. Side effects are rare and limited to headaches, nausea, or irritation at the site of the patch. These symptoms may occur if the patch dose is excessive or can be actually signs of nicotine withdrawal.

Nicotine replacement can also be provided by a special type of chewing gum. Each piece supplies just enough nicotine to avoid withdrawal symptoms. This gum is not like a piece of Bazooka bubble gum. The medicated gum is formulated with resin and is quite tough to chew. When you grind the gum between your teeth, the nicotine separates from the resin and can be absorbed by the bloodstream.

You need to chew nicotine gum differently than you would a piece of Juicy Fruit. It should be chewed just enough to soften it, then tucked between the gum and cheek. You will feel a tingling sensation in your mouth as the nicotine is released. When this happens, you should "park" the gum between your lip and the gum. When the sensation disappears, it is time to chew the gum again to release more nicotine and move the gum to a new location in the mouth.

How much gum you need depends on how many cigarettes a day you usually smoked. If you usually consumed a pack a day, you probably need about ten pieces each day to keep cravings under control. A two pack a day smoker can need as many as twenty pieces to feel comfortable. Over time, you will gradually be able to taper off the amount of gum needed each day. It's not unusual to need nicotine replacement gum for as long as a year to stay an ex-smoker.

The gum may pose a problem if you have jaw or tooth difficulties. It is not like regular chewing gum and can be difficult to chew. If people have any kind of gum or dental problem, they usually cannot tolerate gum. On the plus side, the gum allows you to do something with your hands and your mouth that you normally would be doing with a cigarette. It creates a new ritual by which you can not only wean yourself from the physical withdrawal of cigarettes, but from some of the psychological addictive components as well.

Why Replace One Addiction with Another?

While it is true that nicotine is a noxious substance, and will kill you if you take it in a high enough dose, it is only one of 4,000 different chemicals (including 200 poisons, and 63 known carcinogens) that you inhale with every cigarette puff. If you can prevent these other products from reaching your lungs, by weaning yourself off cigarettes, you may save yourself from many of the health consequences of smoking.

The strategy is to replace the amount of nicotine you use when you smoke by other delivery systems, such as the patch or gum. There are also inhalers or nasal sprays that can be used to deliver nicotine depending on the form you find easiest to use. The advantage of the patch is that one patch lasts twenty-four hours. With all the other strategies, you have to keep re-dosing yourself throughout the day each time you have a craving for a cigarette. That means you might have to use the gum or a spray twenty or thirty times a day, especially in the beginning.

When I am working with someone on smoking cessation, I have to make a judgment about how much nicotine a person is using and start at a compatible level. You don't want to give too much nicotine, because that will make you sick. It is like smoking too much.

Like the recovering alcoholic, the recovering cigarette addict is potentially an addict for life. Through the course of nicotine withdrawal, the various alternative nicotine delivery systems need to be used from three to six months. Keep in mind that you may always be susceptible to starting the habit again. And for that reason, for several years after you quit, it may be a good idea to carry nicotine gum or some other delivery system that you can reach for, rather than reaching for a cigarette.

Be Happy, Stop Smoking

We can also add medication that relieves the depression and anxiety that appears when you try to quit. We use a drug called **Zyban**, which was actually developed as the antidepressant Wellbutrin. In the 1980s, doctors noticed that while treating patients with chronic depression, these people found it easier to stop smoking. This observation led to the use of the drug in smoking cessation trials and it has been shown to be one of the most effective agents we have for helping people quit.

You don't have to be clinically depressed to benefit from **Zyban**. It is the withdrawal of cigarettes, which in effect leads to an *artificial* depression. The absence of smoking creates this lack of anticipation of pleasure, a feeling which mimics depression. If you can't feel like there's something worthwhile in your life, you become depressed and, in somebody who is addicted to cigarettes, it will provoke them to keep smoking.

Zyban is given as a pill. You start out with one of 150 milligrams a day and work up to two tablets a day. **Zyban** is not for everyone. It can cause seizures in people who are predisposed to it. It cannot be used with other antidepressants or antipsychotic agents, or if you are on oral steroids.

Studies have shown that combining **Zyban** and nicotine replacement is about the most effective combination we have to help people stop smoking at this time. Remember, only about one out of ten people who try to quit on their own are successful. With nicotine replacement, that number goes up to 20 or 30 percent. When **Zyban** is used alone, the success rate is 30 to 40 percent. Combining nicotine replacement therapy and **Zyban** can lead up to a 60 percent success rate.

With a Little Help from Your Friends: The Value of Support Groups

Patients often ask me about group programs to help them stop smoking. It is important to remember that the success of smoking cessation is a very individual journey. I have found that for some people it is very reassuring to know that there is a support group or program they could go to, and these patients find a structured program to provide reinforcement from different directions to help them quit. Some of my patients cringe at the idea. I certainly don't want to force someone into a program that upsets them, but for the right person, it can provide emotional and educational support at a critical time and be very useful.

I have found that for smokers who may be somewhat socially isolated, such as widowers or retired people, a smoking support group provides new nonsmoking friends, along with educational, research, and social outlets. Some people find it very reassuring to discuss their addiction with people and to open up to discuss the problems they face.

There are a number of programs available, including "Freedom From Smoking" from the American Lung Association, "Fresh Start" from the American Cancer Society, and the well-known Smokenders. Most of them offer a program of six to eight classes that meet for up to two hours once or twice a week. In a structured, supportive environment, they provide information and motivation. Unfortunately, most groups don't last past the first month and the chances of relapse are greatest in the first three months. But for many people, the program can be there during the first critical weeks of a smoke-free life.

Alternative Treatments

According to a recent Gallup poll more than 20 percent of Americans use nontraditional therapies, such as yoga or herbal remedies, as part of their health care. I have found that my patients have a natural curiosity about the value of the so-called alternative approaches to smoking cessation. Although the studies involving these therapies are often disappointing, it is important to remember that smoking cessation is a personal and unique process. A technique that may not be statistically significant in a study can be invaluable for an individual. I don't discourage my patients from exploring additional support that might be the right step for them.

Hypnosis is one of the oldest types of therapies used to deal with nicotine addiction. It aims to provide posthypnotic suggestions that discourage smoking. Studies have not shown it to be particularly helpful for long-term success. Still, patients have reported to me that, when combined with nicotine replacement therapy, it helps them stay away from cigarettes.

Acupuncture is an ancient Chinese treatment based on the notion that our health is regulated by a series of energy channels that run through the body. Problems arise when blockage occurs to any of these channels. Acupuncture needles are placed at specific points for different problems to relieve these obstructions. Some patients report that needles placed around the ears diminish the side effects of nicotine withdrawal. Unfortunately, there are very few solid studies that show acupuncture works with smoking. As with hypnosis, I suggest that it be used in conjunction, not instead of traditional smoking cessation medication.

Aromatherapy with candles and essential oils is one therapy I would avoid. These fragrances may actually irritate sensitive airways and precipitate wheezing and shortness of breath.

Weight Gain . . . Not Necessarily True

Since the 1980s, we've known that on average people who smoke are about seven to ten pounds lighter than people who don't. This is not something I am happy admitting, but it is true that people who quit smoking gain an average of six to eight pounds. This is a real phenomenon, and it is troubling not only from the perspective of patients in terms of their body image but in terms of their perception of health. Nobody wants to be overweight in this society, and if smoking helps them maintain their weight, it certainly may be an excuse to continue to smoke.

Cigarettes keep weight down in a number of ways. Nicotine is thought to increase metabolism, actually raising the number of calories you burn each day. When you stop smoking, the body metabolism returns to normal. If you don't decrease food intake, you will put on a few pounds. As a stimulant, nicotine also cuts appetite, so you are eating less. When you stop smoking, you eat more and seem to crave sweet and fatty foods. The combination of decreased metabolism and increased appetite leads to the weight gain. That's the bad news. The good news is that nicotine replacement therapy supplies enough nicotine to avoid most of the weight gain. In the three to six months that smokers use the patch and/or gum, they will not gain weight as their body slowly readjusts to a smoke-free status. By the time they cease medication, both appetite and metabolism should have been reset. In fact, 25 percent of people who quit smoking actually lose weight.

Smoking and Exercise

Many heavy smokers are relatively inactive. They find that sports and exercise leave them breathless, and tend to avoid as much activity as possible. They walk rather than run, ride rather than walk, and shudder at the sight of a flight of stairs. When they become ex-smokers, they often join a gym or participate in sports they haven't done since high school. As a result, they lose both pounds and inches.

The Smoking Cessation Strategy

When I start to work with a patient, I tell them to prepare themselves psychologically to quit the day they start the nicotine patch. There is no point continuing smoking and using the patch. In fact, it is probably harmful because you will be getting a double dose of nicotine. On the other hand, with **Zyban**, you need a week to build up a level of medication in your blood that allows you to withdraw comfortably from cigarettes. I begin my smoking cessation program by giving my patient a week on **Zyban**. At this point, they are still smoking, but they will notice they will want fewer cigarettes. After about a week on the antidepressant when the blood levels are high, I add a nicotine patch. In addition, I have them carry nicotine gum or a spray to give them an extra lift during the day if they feel a sudden craving. This treatment continues two to three months. My patients are monitored closely and call me every week to report how they are doing.

Alcohol and Smoking

Many of the psychological reasons that cause people to become addicted cut across the substances they use. There are psychological and physiological reasons for addiction and it is not unusual to see multiple addictions in the same person. We know that many drug addicts are inveterate smokers, and it's not surprising to have one, two, or three addictive substances used simultaneously. This situation creates difficult strategy problems for both the patient and the doctor.

Patients who have an alcohol problem in addition to smoking ask me if they should try to quit both at the same time. This needs to be handled on an individual basis. I have been told that it is much easier to quit alcohol than smoking, and so a step-wise approach might be appropriate. On the other hand, for the individual who goes into a program like a structured rehabilitation environment, it may be possible to quit more than one addiction, such as alcohol and drugs, at the same time. In general, this is a very difficult time to quit cigarettes. I would suggest that, if you have pulmonary problems, you should tackle the smoking problem first. Get that under control, then deal with other issues.

The Gift That Keeps on Giving

Devoting the time and energy to smoking cessation is one of the best presents you can give yourself. Within just a few weeks, you will notice a difference in the way you feel. Within a few weeks, unhealthy high blood pressure readings can begin to drop. Within a year, heart disease death rate is halfway back to that of a nonsmoker. After five years nonsmoking, the risk of oral and esophageal cancers is cut in half. In a study conducted at the University of Utah, researchers reported that within five years of quitting, people had improved lung function, less coughing, and reduced shortness of breath. For a former smoker, the numbers just keep getting better and better.

Chapter 9

Treatment Strategies for Asthma and COPD

"Tell me the truth, Dr. Schachter, is my sister dying?" said my caller, his voice shaking with concern. "She came to see you for a cough and left your office with five prescriptions." I hastened to assure Harry O'Brien that his sister had easily controllable asthma and that the different prescriptions would work on different aspects of the asthmatic process to keep her symptom-free.

Different Drugs for Different Problems

There are at least six distinct categories of medications that are routinely used for asthma/COPD and each offers unique benefits. While it can be alarming to suddenly see a row of pills and inhalers on your nightstand, it is more a reflection of what we have learned about the causes of airway obstruction than a sign of the seriousness of your illness. Symptoms arise through a host of different mechanisms, and each classification of drugs addresses these problems in a unique way.

Bronchodilators—The Ties That Unbind

Bronchodilators do exactly what their name implies. They dilate or widen constricted airways. There are two major types of bronchodilators and each acts on separate receptor sites on the cells that make the airways narrow. Receptor sites are keyhole-like structures on the outside surface of the cell that allow chemicals such as hormones to "lock" onto the cell and affect cellular activity. For example, when adrenalin locks onto its receptor site on heart and blood vessel muscle, it can increase heart rate and raise blood pressure. Manipulating or blocking adrenalin receptor sites with beta blockers is a strategy we use for everyday control of blood pressure.

Here's how it works in the lungs: The smooth muscle of our airways is dotted with what we call beta 2 receptors. As you will remember from Chapter 5, smooth muscle is the active part of the airways that gives these structures their tone. These muscles allow the airways to adopt a shape and size so that they do not collapse during the normal act of breathing. Under abnormal circumstances (such as an asthmatic attack), these smooth muscles contract excessively, causing airways to shrink, making breathing difficult. We use beta agonists to activate these beta 2 receptor sites, causing the smooth muscle to relax, thereby preventing or reversing this process, in other words, relaxing tightened airways. Researchers have been able to tailor bronchodilators to act on these beta 2 receptors so that they are as specific as possible thereby limiting side effects.

Short-acting beta agonists begin working within seconds, but the effects last minutes to a few hours. As a result, you can feel the difference in your breathing almost instantly. For practical purposes, we use a period of ten minutes to evaluate the full extent of the activity of the short-acting beta agonists, but, in fact, most of their effect is seen within just one or two minutes. If problems are due primarily to simple bronchospasm, a puff or two from a beta agonist inhaler will relieve your shortness of breath.

Beta agonists are not without their problems. We try to design these drugs to be as specific as possible for the relaxing receptors on the airway smooth muscle. Unfortunately, it is not possible to make these drugs totally specific. This means that other beta receptors get activated, causing side effects that include increased heart rate, palpitation, muscle tremors, and a sense of nervousness. In some people, this can progress to an irregular heartbeat and an abnormal heart rhythm.

Short-acting beta agonists can be the only medication you need for mild intermittent asthma with infrequent and limited symptoms. Beta agonists can be carried as a "rescue medication," used at those infrequent times when wheezing or coughing develop. We also use short-acting beta agonists for additional help if you have a more severe form of lung obstruction and are subject to frequent unexpected attacks. Problems arise when you use these short-acting drugs too frequently. If your symptoms are too severe to be controlled by occasional use, or your airways are no longer responding to this medication, you need additional treatment. You can find yourself in a medical crisis due to life-threatening side effects following overuse, or acute respiratory failure if the medication no longer relieves your symptoms. This tragic consequence occurred in 1995 when model Christy Taylor died from asthma attributed to overuse of this type of short-acting drug.

Examples of effective short-acting beta agonists include **Ventolin, Albuterol, Alupent,** or **Proventil.** They are usually administered as a spray in a metered-dose inhaler known as an MDI: a canister which contains the liquid medicine under pressure. When you squeeze the MDI inhaler, the spray is released and you inhale it into your lungs in a fixed amount, so we know exactly how much medicine was given. Another delivery system commonly used for this type of medication is the aerosol nebulizer. This requires a special instrument that creates a mist that is inhaled through a mouthpiece or face mask.

For mild asthma or bronchitis, you may require only one or two doses of a short-acting bronchodilator to feel comfortable throughout the day. Some of my patients with mild asthma use it on a weekly or even on a monthly basis. But when your airways are constricted almost all the time, you will need a longer-acting medication such as **Serevent,** which is taken more regularly.

Essentially, these long-acting agents work in much the same way as the short-acting forms, in that they act on the beta 2 receptor and cause airway smooth muscle to relax. The major difference is that the effect of the long-acting beta agonist lasts between eight and twelve hours. It becomes a medication that can be used twice daily instead of four or five times a day to control persistent symptoms.

The long-acting beta agonists tend to have a slower onset of action and it may take twenty to sixty minutes before the relief is apparent. When people first use them, they don't notice their bronchial dilating effects as dramatically as they do with short-acting beta agonists. But bear with it, because within a day or so, you should experience a great sense of long-term comfort and relief. Patients have told me that using a long-acting beta agonist twice a day makes them forget that they have respiratory problems. The long-acting beta agonists provide sustained relief for breathing, unlike the short-acting agents, which peak early but cannot maintain their effect over several hours. Long-acting beta agonists have the same side effects as short-acting medications, including nervousness and tremors, but in general the side effects are less troublesome.

For many of my patients with asthma/COPD, I prescribe both types of beta agonists. The long-acting beta agonist is used to establish an improved bronchial state through the day, whereas the short-acting beta agonist is used as a rescue medication. For example, if you decide to run for a bus in cold weather, you may suddenly get short of breath, even though you used your long-acting beta agonist. That's when one to two puffs of the short-acting beta agonist inhaler will provide quick relief. Short-acting beta agonists can also be used to prevent problems. If you are invited to dinner at the home of a friend who is a cat owner, two puffs on the inhaler before you arrive can stabilize your airways and prevent or minimize an asthmatic attack.

Same Game, Different Play

A second group of bronchodilators known as anticholinergic work by blocking the effect of acetylcholine on the airways. Acetylcholine is a mediator released by the vagus nerve which branches into the airways and controls the tone of the smooth muscle in the bronchial tree. The regulation of airway tone is but one of the many functions of acetylcholine. It is a ubiquitous neural mediator responsible for digestive function, heart rate, and vision.

The original anticholinergic drug has been around for centuries. It was known as belladonna, because it was used as an eyedrop that caused the pupil of the eye to dilate and gave Roman women a very dark and mysterious look to their eyes. While cosmetically interesting, this may not be something you would want in a medication. Not only does it open the pupil and make your eye darker, but it paralyzes the muscle that allows you to focus. You may look very beautiful, but you can't see who you're with.

The older anticholinergic medication was used relatively sparingly in respiratory medicine because the cholinergic nervous system affects so many organs that the use of these drugs produced a host of unwanted side effects, including fast heart rate and blurred vision. In addition, the original anticholinergics were very short-acting. Today the modern anticholinergic drug **Atrovent,** delivered by an inhaler, prevents the absorption and widespread action seen with older anticholinergic medications that limited their effectiveness and safety in the treatment of the pulmonary system.

This class of drugs is used in treating lung disease because the cholinergic nervous system operates the nerves in the airways that give the airways their tone. When these nerves in the airways are activated by the cholinergic system, they cause airway smooth muscle to contract. Anticholinergic inhaled drugs, such as **Atrovent** and the soon to be released **Spireva**, act on the vagus nerve and prevent this constriction. Spireva will have the very great advantage over Atrovent (a short-acting drug) in that Spireva will be a long-acting, once-a-day agent.

Spireva is currently approved for the treatment of COPD in several European countries and is being considered by the FDA here in the United States. Anecdotal reports from patients as well as preliminary publications indicate that Spireva is safe and makes a noticeable improvement in the quality of life of patients with COPD.

Like beta agonists, anticholinergic drugs work on specific receptor sites. They act by blocking the cholinergic receptors on airway smooth muscle. This action is independent of the smooth muscle relaxing activity of beta drugs. Anticholinergic therapy has proven particularly effective for patients with classic COPD (chronic bronchitis and emphysema). When we combine an anticholinergic drug and beta agonists, such as in the drug **Combivent**, we modulate both receptors and provide even better bronchodilating relief for patients, enhancing the degree of impact. Happily, the combination of both drugs has no more side effects than either one of the medications taken separately.

Controlling the Source of the Problems: Anti-Inflammatory Drugs

Inflammation is the driving force behind sustained airway obstruction. We have now come to realize that controlling this inflammation is the best tool we have for both symptom relief and prevention of permanent lung damage and airway remodeling. In order to understand why it is so important to control this inflammation, I want to explain what inflammation does to your body. If you touch a poison ivy plant, your skin becomes swollen, red, and itchy. That reaction mimics the inflammatory response that we can see on a microscopic level inside the body tissues. Inflammation makes blood vessels leak, attracts white blood cells to the area so they can respond to the threatening agents, and causes smooth muscles to constrict.

When you give anti-inflammatory drugs, you reverse this process. You stop fluid oozing from the blood vessels, you prevent the migration of white blood cells, and you relax the constriction of smooth muscles and calm overactivity of the mucous glands.

The Drug My Patients Love to Hate

When corticosteroids were first introduced in 1948, they were hailed as a miracle drug. For the first time, doctors had a single, inexpensive drug that could relieve a wide range of serious problems. It enabled a wheelchair-bound arthritic to walk with ease. Patients with lupus found that their joint, kidney, and skin problems seemingly disappeared. It gave people with nephritis, a serious kidney disorder, a new lease on life. In the emergency room, cortisone reduced life-threatening swelling and allergic reactions. Their impact was so remarkable that the three doctors who pioneered cortisone research were awarded the Nobel Prize for Medicine in 1950.

The ink was scarcely dry on their award when reports of problems began to flood the medical journals. It turned out that the miracle drug carried a very heavy price tag. Over time, patients treated with cortisone developed fragile bones, diabetes, and life-threatening infections. The image of cortisone changed from the great discovery of the twentieth century to a symbol of the dark side of medicine.

The hunt began for a form of steroid therapy that would have good anti-inflammatory effects, but few or none of the bad side effects. One of the earliest strategies was to give oral steroids every other day, but this strategy was only partly successful. In fact, many people did not get enough benefits from the alternate day steroids and still experienced unacceptable levels of side effects.

The breakthrough for airway disease came when potent aerosol treatment with steroids became available. With these aerosol treatments, it became possible to concentrate high doses of the drug just on the airways without flooding steroids throughout the rest of the body. There are a number of effective steroid inhalers, including **Flovent, Pulmicort, AeroBid, Azmacort,** and **Vanceril.** Most commonly, you would take two to four puffs a day. Studies have repeatedly demonstrated the value of inhaled steroids. These include reducing the frequency of asthma attacks and making the airway less irritable, thereby reducing symptoms.

Each year more than 500,000 Americans are admitted to hospitals due to asthma and more than 5,000 children and adults with asthma die. A study published in the *New England Journal of Medicine* reported that even low doses of inhaled corticosteroids reduced the risk of death by half. Similarly, a Canadian study of 22,000 people with COPD found that after one year, those using inhaled corticosteroids had a 24 percent lower hospitalization rate. Even more encouraging, those on steroids had a 29 percent lower mortality rate.

Most patients on aerosol steroids can take them for long periods of time with relatively few side effects. With inhaled steroids, the problems are usually local. They include soreness of the mouth and tongue, hoarseness of the throat, and a local infection known as thrush. All of these side effects can be handled by relatively simple strategies, such as rinsing out your mouth and gargling after you have used the inhaled steroids. You can also use a spacer, which allows the aerosol to be inhaled without precipitating into the upper airway. Accumulation of steroid on the tongue or in the throat can lead to a sore throat or sore mouth or even *thrush,* a topical fungal infection with candida. Some people develop hoarseness as a result of this deposition.

Aerosol steroids may still affect other areas of the body. A study published in the *New England Journal of Medicine* followed 100 women aged eighteen to forty-five who used steroid inhalers. At the end of three years, researchers found that women had lost bone density. The more steroids they used, the greater bone loss they experienced. Other studies have reported some degree of loss in bone density, but not an increase in fractures or osteoporosis. As yet, we don't know the clinical significance of these bone changes, but we do know the consequences of untreated inflammation of the airways. At this point in time, inhaled steroids are the best way we have to prevent progressive and irreversible airway disease. By contrast, we have a number of tools to deal with bone density concerns. Overall, the use of chronic inhaled steroid therapy is remarkably well tolerated and most physicians, following their clinical experience as well as national guidelines, use these treatments extensively for the control of moderate to severe asthma, as well as in mild persistent asthma.

To avoid problems, I have referred high-risk patients for bone density tests if they have been on inhaled steroids for more than two years. In addition, I am now recommending calcium intake of 1,200 mg/day, from a combination of diet and supplements, and urging at-risk patients to do weight bearing exercises that build bones. In women with a personal or family history of osteoporosis, I might recommend a bone-building medication such as **Fosamax,** and referral to a metabolism specialist.

There have also been some anecdotal reports about an increased risk of cataracts with inhaled steroids. A recent retrospective study from Boston University School of Medicine found that there was a very slight increase in risk of cataracts for people over forty using inhaled corticosteroids. Younger patients had no problems with cataract development.

The effectiveness of aerosol steroids for chronic bronchitis and emphysema has been questioned because it is felt the inflammation that causes the progressive disease is different from that which causes the damage in asthma. The white blood cells associated with asthmatic inflammation are frequently the eosinophils, and that type of inflammation responds very well to corticosteroids. In chronic bronchitis and emphysema, the white blood cells are more frequently neutrophils, which appear to be less sensitive to corticosteroids.

This does not mean that steroids are ineffective for chronic obstructive pulmonary disease. Between 15 and 25 percent of COPD patients respond well to steroids, and we suspect that many of them have elements of both asthma and COPD. Interestingly, when COPD patients become ill with acute exacerbations, they respond very well to steroids, and almost invariably require them.

There are different preparations and different means of delivering corticosteroids. They can be injected directly into the veins, under the skin, or deep into the muscles. I can also prescribe steroids in pill as well as aerosol form. Each of these routes has their advantages and disadvantages. The injectable form is probably most useful for very sick, acutely ill patients with COPD and/or asthma. In these situations, you want to deliver a high dose very rapidly, and the best way to do that is either intravenously or intramuscularly. For patients with moderately severe disease or dealing with an acute exacerbation, Prednisone, a steroid in pill form, may be necessary for a week to ten days. We don't want to keep people on oral steroids for any longer than we have to, because there are side effects.

Most patients with lung disease get them in the form of aerosol, and there are two ways they can be delivered. One is in a true aerosol spray, which is wet and is inhaled from a metered-dose inhaler (MDI). These sprays, such as **Flovent** and **AeroBid,** can deliver a single, accurate dose at a time.

There is a second form of these aerosol corticosteroids, such as **Pulmicort,** which is in the form of a dry powder. These are also delivered by an inhaler, but instead of being sprayed as a jet of droplets, the powder is inhaled and absorbed on the surface of the lungs. **Advair** is an inhaled powder that combines a corticosteroid (**Flovent**) with a long-acting bronchodilator (**Serevent**).

This type of combination therapy has proven very effective in reducing asthma symptoms and attacks and in improving patient compliance. The multi-dose **Diskus** is particularly simple to use. Another version of this form of combination therapy, **Symbicort** is available in Europe, combining **Pulmicort** (a corticosteroid) and **Formoterol** (a long-acting beta agonist). It is currently in clinical trials here in the United States.

Asthma Treatments for Children—Similar but Separate

Treatment guidelines from the National Heart Blood and Lung Institute (NHLBI) have recently (2002) been updated to reflect new insights into the dynamics of asthma in childhood. Because it is difficult for children under the age of six to use an inhaler, aerosol medication is delivered via a nebulizer, a device which produces a fine mist that is released into a face mask or a mouthpiece. A parent needs to place the face mask over the child's nose and mouth, switch on the device, and the child then inhales the medication by breathing normally.

For infants and toddlers, this can be more difficult than it sounds. Very young children often fight off the mask and it can be a daily battle between the wheezy child and the frantic parents. Holding the small child on your lap and trying to make the nebulizer into a game can help ensure that their lungs get the relief they need.

Generally, children do not respond as well as adults to bronchodilators. To keep airways open, doctors now use aerosolized steroids to reduce inflammation. There has been some concern that steroids slow a child's growth, but the latest studies show that a slowdown in growth is usually only temporary and most children eventually catch up in height.

In addition to steroids, pediatric pulmonologists recommend two additional types of medication: chromones such as **Intal**, which act by preventing the release of mediators, such as histamine, from airway mast cells. These mediators are the chemicals that play an important role in the allergic reaction. These medications are rarely used in adults but can be effective in childhood, where allergies are the driving force behind asthmatic attacks.

Leukotriene blocking agents, such as **Singulair**, are very popular because they can be given as a pill or a liquid. Not only do they seem to be more effective in children, but the ease of delivery makes life simpler for parents and child. They act by blocking the attachment of leukotrienes to their cell receptors, a reaction that would otherwise cause swelling, mucus production in the airways, and bronchoconstriction.

Although asthma in children can be dramatic and frightening, the good news is that more than 50 percent of children with asthma seem to outgrow their disease by the time they reach their teens. For many, it may never appear again. For others, it can be provoked by exposure to irritants in adulthood. If symptoms do recur, it is important to get a proper diagnosis and appropriate treatment. Adults respond well to bronchodilators and should include this type of medication as part of any asthma regimen.

Preventing Respiratory Problems

Anything that we can do to prevent, halt, or limit respiratory infection in people with asthma/COPD prevents irreversible airway damage. Infection causes high levels of inflammation, as well as a breakdown of your pulmonary tissue. The enzymes that are released by the white blood cells that arrive to combat infection are able to destroy the network of connective tissues that maintains the functional structure of the lung. Consequently, anyone with pulmonary disease must start off autumn with a flu shot. Because the type of virus that causes influenza changes on a yearly basis, you need to be immunized against the current virus every year.

There are also medications available to decrease the severity and length of time of a viral infection once it is established, but the best way to avoid the damage of the flu is to prevent it. If the flu does occur (and no vaccine is 100 percent effective), then antiviral drugs can play a role in limiting symptoms and possibly lung damage. Medications such as **Tamiflu** can reduce the severity and length of influenza. To be effective, they should be given within thirty-six hours of infection and taken for five to ten days. These medications should not be used if you are pregnant or breastfeeding.

Are Flu Vaccines Safe If I Have Asthma?

Concerns have been raised that flu shots can exacerbate asthma symptoms. A beautifully designed nationwide study sponsored by the American Lung Association and published recently in the *New England Journal of Medicine* has put these fears to rest. The well-controlled crossover study of 2,000 people with asthma found that the rate of asthma attacks were equal in asthmatics given flu vaccines and those receiving a placebo.

We also have a vaccination against specific forms of bacterial pneumonia caused by pneumococcus. Unlike vaccines that protect against only one or two strains of flu virus, the pneumonia vaccine protects against over twenty different strains of these bacteria. Even better, the pneumonia vaccine is known to be effective for five to ten years. There are some side effects from the pneumonia vaccine similar to those from a flu shot, including local redness, headache, and perhaps a touch of fever. I make sure that all of my pulmonary patients are protected with both the flu and pneumonia vaccine.

Antibiotics for a Cold?

When antibiotics were first discovered, they were used for everything. Over the years, we stopped using antibiotics for viral infections such as colds and flus because antibiotics have no impact on viruses. But when you have pulmonary disease, antibiotics play a very important protective role when colds and flus develop. We don't want to abuse antibiotics because there are downsides to overuse: You can develop side effects, allergic reactions, and cause bacteria to become resistant. On the other hand, in people with COPD a simple cold, or flu, or even sinus infection can lead to big problems. I will frequently tell my patients with chronic obstructive lung disease to take antibiotics at the first sign of a chest cold.

We have a number of different classes of antibiotics to choose from and we want to select one that is effective against common bacteria associated with COPD. There are four main categories of antibiotics: *beta lactams*, such as penicillin (and its derivatives such as amoxicillin), kill bacteria by inhibiting cell wall synthesis. The first class of antibiotics to be discovered, penicillins are generally inexpensive and can be effective against a wide range of organisms. When they work, these antibiotics can quickly bring a severe infection under control. Unfortunately, a significant number of people have developed allergies to them. In addition, we have seen the rise of penicillin-resistant strains of bacteria that are found in respiratory infections. One form of resistance involves the bacterial production of an enzyme that renders the antibiotic ineffective. This can be overcome by combining the beta lactam with a chemical such as clavulinic acid. The combination of amoxicillin and clavulinic acid **(Augmentin)** can enhance the killing power of the beta lactams.

Another form of beta lactam antibiotic is called cephalosporins (such as **Ceftin** and **Ceclor**). For many bacteria that cause respiratory infections, cephalosporins are as effective as penicillins. Because of the similarity in molecular structure, patients with recent major penicillin allergies should not be given cephalosporins. Those persons with lesser allergies should take these medications with caution. Like penicillin, a number of cephalosporin-resistant strains of bacteria have now appeared.

Macrolides are a class of antibiotics that includes **Zithromax, Biaxin,** and **Erythromycin.** They are bacteriostatic, meaning they don't kill bacteria but slow them down by inhibiting their metabolism (protein synthesis). They work well against organisms such as streptococcus that cause pneumonia, but unlike the beta lactam antibiotics, they are also effective against less common agents such as mycoplasma and legionella, which can cause serious infections in patients with respiratory disease. Macrolides are well tolerated and can be used safely if you have an allergy to penicillin. As with beta lactams, there are now macrolide-resistant bacteria, but resistance is less of a problem than with beta lactams.

Fluoroquinolones are a very effective class of antibiotics usually reserved for very sick patients when other antibiotics have failed to control infection. They kill bacteria by disrupting their DNA strands. This relatively new class of antibiotics became front-page news when the fluoroquinolone **Cipro** was named as the drug of choice for anthrax. Other fluoroquinolones include **Levaquin, Tequin,** and **Avelox.** One of the reasons that they work so well is that few resistant strains have yet appeared—and we want to keep it that way. The best way to do that is to avoid overuse, when older antibiotics would be equally effective. Fluoroquinolones are expensive and can occasionally have serious side effects, but it is reassuring to know that they are available when necessary.

Tetracyclines are bacteriostatic antibiotics that inhibit bacterial protein synthesis. They have a very broad range of activity against both gram positive and gram negative bacteria, the two major classes of bacteria that cause respiratory infections, as well as mycoplasma, legionella, and chlamydia. Inexpensive and well tolerated, their effectiveness has been compromised by drug-resistant strains of bacteria.

Selecting an Antibiotic

For simple bronchitis in a healthy individual, treatment may not require an antibiotic as many of these illnesses are caused by viruses. For patients with simple chronic bronchitis who develop an exacerbation with a bronchial infection, a tetracycline, a macrolide, or a beta lactam antibiotic is usually sufficient. Courses are usually five to seven days. In patients with complicated chronic bronchitis (age greater than sixty-five, more than four episodes a year, and with abnormal pulmonary function and/or associated serious diseases such as heart disease) who develop an exacerbation with a bronchial infection, fluoroquinolones or the enhanced beta lactams (such as **Augmentin**) are usually effective in curing the infection and restoring better lung function.

Mediator-Modifying Drugs

Up to this point, we have talked about drugs that are prescribed for asthma, as well as for chronic bronchitis and emphysema. In addition, there are drugs that are specifically effective for asthma alone, targeting factors related to the inflammation unique to hypersensitive airways.

Antihistamines that are commonly used for upper respiratory airway symptoms like sinusitis, rhinitis (runny nose), or hay fever may relieve or prevent allergy-provoked asthma. These drugs act by blocking the effects of histamine, which is a mediator that causes the blood vessels to swell and leak and that stimulates white blood cells to migrate to the area of inflammation. While antihistamines are not that effective in reducing bronchospasm, they can relieve upper airway congestion that may trigger airways to constrict.

A new group of controller agents affects leukotrienes, the mediators released in an allergy-induced cascade. Drugs such as **Accolate** and **Singulair** inhibit the synthesis of leukotrienes or block their action on the receptors. Remember that mucus production, bronchoconstriction, and swelling are provoked by the action of leukotrienes. These medications are easy to use, have few side effects, and need to be taken only once or twice a day in pill form. They work primarily for highly allergic asthmatics, but are less effective than inhaled steroids and bronchodilators for most patients.

Another group of drugs, known as chromones, block the release of mediators from the mast cells, and can be particularly effective in allergic inflammation in children. **Intal** is taken using an inhaler or a nebulizer, a machine that takes a liquid dispersion and aerosolizes it. In other words, it makes it into tiny droplets that contain active medication. This is powered by a stream of air that pushes the fine particles into the airways. When you inhale, the particles of medication are spread through the airways, settling down on these sensitive cells.

There are a growing number of mediators (like histamine and leukotrienes) as well as cytokines (natural body secretions that attract inflammatory cells to areas of injury) that have been identified with inflammation. Research has led to design new agents which specifically inhibit these mediators or cytokines. Perhaps one of the most novel approaches is a new agent with the difficult to pronounce name of **Omaluzimab** (to be known as **Xolair** when it is approved). Unlike the mediator specific drugs it is an anti-antibody which specifically targets and blocks immunoglobulin E (IgE) the antibody which turns on many allergic cells such as the mast cell and basophil cell making them release mediators. Treatment with this anti-antibody can virtually eliminate IgE from the blood for two to four weeks. Preliminary clinical testing has been very encouraging, reducing the frequency of asthma attacks. It does have to be given by injection and is at this time a very expensive treatment, but one with promise.

Can't You Just Give Me Something for This Cough?

Many patients who come to me are looking for the ultimate cough syrup. But coughing is the way the body clears the lungs of mucus, dirt, and irritants. Rather than prescribing a medication to suppress the cough, I look at the issues that are causing it.

The three most common causes for persistent cough are: 1) Cough variant asthma; 2) Chronic sinus or upper respiratory tract infection; and surprisingly 3) Acid reflux from the stomach, which may or may not be associated with obvious heartburn.

There are basically three types of cough syrups:

Cough suppressants (also known as antitussives) inhibit

activity in the brain that controls the cough reflex. Prescription cough suppressants contain codeine, while those that are available over the counter are formulated with dextromethorphan. I prescribe these primarily if a cough is keeping you up at night.

Expectorants thin and loosen mucus secretions. Available without a prescription, the active ingredient in these products is guaifenesin. This type of cough syrup may loosen a dry, unproductive cough, and help you bring up mucus, but have little value for coughs due to asthma/COPD.

Combination cough syrup contains a mix of suppressants, expectorants, antihistamines, decongestants, and aspirin. This shotgun approach may help relieve cold and flu symptoms for healthy lungs.

Still the bottom line is that I want to see your cough controlled by dealing with the underlying inflammation and bronchoconstriction, rather than simply masking the symptom with narcotics. That being said, sometimes it is important to control coughing. For example, when the coughing prevents the patient from sleeping, or the cough perpetuates airway irritability, I may prescribe a cough medication to be used along with your other specific medications, not in place of them.

Everything Old Is New Again

Theophylline is a medication that belongs to a group of drugs known as the methylxanthines. Probably the best known of these types of medications is caffeine, which is the active ingredient in coffee. Originally, theophylline was valued for its ability to relax the muscles in the airways. In other words, like beta agonists and anticholinergics, theophylline acts as a bronchodilator. It also has several unique properties. It can be given as a pill, a liquid, an elixir, or by injection. It is a very effective medication for the treatment of airway obstruction and, for a long time, it was the number one drug used for the treatment of these conditions. It fell out of favor in the 1990s, primarily because of its side effects. Unlike many other medications that we use, the side effects unfortunately seemed to occur at exactly the same level where the beneficial effects appeared. In other words, it had a very narrow therapeutic to toxic ratio. Just when you were actually breathing easier, most of the really bad side effects appeared.

The impact was often quite individual, and some people were more sensitive than others. But just about everyone who took a high enough dose would experience nausea, vomiting, nervousness, sleeplessness, and occasionally much more severe side effects, such as heart arrhythmias or seizures. The fact that such bad things could happen with such a good drug made most physicians drop it from their pulmonary armamentarium. However, it has now made a modest resurgence in usage because we are discovering not only how better to use it, but how many ways it can be beneficial, particularly in chronic obstructive lung disease.

One of the things that we have learned is that theophylline has the ability to increase the strength of the diaphragm. Remember, that is the muscle that separates the lungs from the abdomen and, for healthy people, accounts for most of the efforts that we exert to breathe. For patients with chronic obstructive lung disease where there is an overinflation of the lungs, the diaphragm may be in a position where it works inefficiently and tires easily. A drug that can enhance the strength of the diaphragm can be very desirable.

We also have realized that the theophylline levels we used were much too high. We now know that when they are combined with other bronchodilators, we can get the benefits from theophylline at much lower doses than we thought previously possible. It turns out that theophylline works additively with beta agonists and anticholinergic drugs, complementing their benefits and adding a few of their own. Today I use theophylline to control difficult to manage symptoms, particularly when other medications lose their effectiveness.

Theophylline works in part by blocking an enzyme in the body's cells known as phosphodiesterase. This enzyme is found widely in cells throughout the body and may account for many side effects of theophylline. A new class of agents known as phosphodiesterase IV inhibitors is being evaluated because it is felt that these medications will have fewer side effects than theophylline and potentially may be more effective. Preliminary experience with agents like **Ariflo** has been encouraging.

Blending Eastern and Western Medicine

I met Judy Jacobson at an Earth Day Celebration, where our daughters manned a "Save Our Earth" booth together. Smart, intense, and very funny, Judy long held an interest in alternative, especially Eastern, medical therapies. She was justifiably proud of her ongoing good health and loved sending me homeopathic remedies for my annual winter cold.

When she developed environmental asthma after her Woodstock home was flooded, she turned to herbal remedies to relieve her breathing problems. When these tinctures and teas failed to control her symptoms, Judy allowed her husband to drag her to their family physician, and she was horrified when he prescribed oral steroids. Angry and in tears, she called me for help. We sat down together to work out a treatment plan that made us both feel comfortable, one that **combined** alternative and conservative medical strategies.

When patients like Judy want to use nontraditional therapies, I believe that it is important to explain the strengths and weaknesses of these treatments and determine the ways they can be utilized. Judy was particularly interested in acupuncture and there is a considerable amount of research on the role of this ancient Chinese remedy in asthma treatment.

Acupuncture is the traditional form of Chinese medicine that relies on "readjusting the balance of energies between organs." Practitioners of acupuncture have mapped median lines and points in the body, and stimulate these areas with fine needles to control disease and relieve symptoms. Research has shown that acupuncture needles at the "Din Chuan point" on the back can relieve bronchoconstriction as effectively as a low dose of a short-acting inhaled bronchodilator. The effect is short-lived and there is concern that, although acupuncture can reduce a sense of breathlessness, it has no effect on inflammation. In China, acupuncture is used along with the more traditional Western medicine and not as the sole therapy. If you want to explore acupuncture, use it in concert with prescribed medications and monitor the effects of treatments with your handheld peak flow meter. With this technique, Judy was able to see how much relief she was getting from acupuncture and when she needed additional support from bronchodilators.

Herbal treatment for asthma is almost as old as the practice of medicine. As we saw, belladonna from the nightshade plant had been used for centuries to relieve shortness of breath. Ma-Huang, a Chinese herb still used today, contains ephedrine, a chemical closely related to adrenalin. Unfortunately, there are few standards for the strength and purity of herbal preparations found in health food stores and Chinese pharmacies. The quality can vary from useless to dangerous. Some so-called natural products are "juiced up" with theophylline or steroids to make them seem more effective, but these ingredients are not listed on the label. It is easy to take doses that are too weak to help, or too strong, resulting in serious side effects. While the idea of herbs may seem more naturally healthy than a plastic canister of bronchodilator, it is important to remember that both have the same class of chemicals, but the inhaler delivers a measured and consistent dose of medication.

The Mind/Body Connection in Asthma

It is clear that shortness of breath in asthma/COPD can be triggered and exacerbated by anxiety and stress. Because tranquilizers and antidepressants can also depress the respiratory system, leading to reduced ventilation and even respiratory failure, doctors have looked to relaxation strategies such as yoga, biofeedback, and hypnosis. While no single technique has been proven unilaterally effective, there are enough anecdotal reports to warrant a closer look.

Yoga is the old Sanskrit word meaning "yoke" or "union," signifying a state of harmony for mind and body. There are a number of different types of yoga, which use varying combinations of exercise, meditation, and breathing techniques. Studies have shown that healthy people who practice yoga have lowered breathing rates and increased lung capacity. Other health benefits reported include a decrease in blood pressure, reduction in chronic pain, and decline in stress levels.

Yoga breathing exercises called *pranayamas* are designed to prepare the mind to relax. When we are tense, we take shallow irregular breaths. *Pranayamas* emphasize inhaling through the nostrils, rather than the mouth. This allows the air to be warmed and filtered of pollutants and allergens through the nasal passages before reaching the lungs. Good posture is equally important for yogic breathing control. When your shoulders are slumped or rounded, the rib cage presses on the diaphragm, limiting chest expansion. The straight upright position of the *pranayamas* promotes full, healthy expansion of the chest during respiration.

Yoga practice cannot substitute for your medication, but can be used in conjunction with your prescribed treatment program. Although their FEV1 remained unchanged, patients have reported fewer symptoms and an improved quality of life when they do yoga.

Meditation is another time-honored relaxation technique. Though it originated centuries ago in the Far East, Western medicine has only recently begun to explore its health benefits. Studies from Harvard by Dr. Herbert Benson demonstrated that transcendental meditation (TM) could reduce blood pressure, lower stress hormone levels, and slow heart rate. Meditation also lowers oxygen needs of the body, an important benefit if you have obstructive lung disease. There are books, audio-tapes, and videos that can introduce and guide you to TM techniques. If you are interested, check in your community for classes and programs that offer meditation instruction.

Although published studies have not conclusively demonstrated meditation benefits, some of my patients report that they feel better and have fewer acute episodes when TM is added to their treatment plan. Since anxiety and stress are well-known triggers for lung disease, anything that can reduce negative factors is certainly a step in the right direction.

Teaching Your Body to Relax

Biofeedback is a scientific way to learn control of autonomic activity, such as heart rate and muscle tension. During a biofeedback session, sensitive equipment monitors one or more body functions, such as skin temperature or blood pressure. Then, using your stress reduction techniques such as TM or yoga, you consciously try to regulate body activity. Depending on how they are used, biofeedback monitors can register changes in blood pressure, tension, and heart rate as you focus on relaxing body activities.

To help you "learn" to relax, sensors are painlessly attached to your body to record muscle tension or pulse rate. A small machine about the size of a portable TV will record impulses from your body. These findings will register either as a quick bleep or a flashing light. For example, if your goal is to lower your heart rate, a light may turn from red to green when your pulse rate drops below seventy. This trains your body to respond to relaxation techniques. The goal is to master exercises without needing the feedback from laboratory equipment.

In my practice, I have found that relaxation strategies work best in people with flexible schedules. Patients who are working and caring for a family find it difficult and actually stressful to commit to taking the time for TM or yoga. People who are retired, or those with fewer family commitments, actually enjoy the opportunity to explore something new and potentially beneficial. If you do choose to include relaxation techniques, remember they are to be used in conjunction with, not instead of, daily medications.

Putting Theory into Practice

With all these categories of drugs and therapies, your doctor can tailor a treatment program depending on your needs. If you have very mild intermittent asthma, he or she might just start you off with a short-acting beta agonist to be used as rescue medication to either prevent a problem when you know you're coming into a high-trigger situation or to use if problems develop unexpectedly. It is important, however, to make sure that you carry your inhaler with you continually. Replace it before its expiration date, and check each morning that it is in good working condition. A study published in *Pulmonary Pediatrics* showed that 30 percent of asthma fatalities occurred in mild forms of asthma, and it's felt that it's partially due to the fact that these people were simply not carrying the medication they needed.

If the severity and frequency of your asthma symptoms increase, your doctor would add additional medications. If you have persistent, even mild persistent symptoms, he or she would probably start you on three medications: an anti-inflammatory drug to bring the inflammation under control; a long-acting beta agonist; and a short-acting rescue inhaler to be used if needed.

As discussed, many patients tend to be reluctant to use a steroid. Doctors have even given this attitude its own name, "Steroid Phobia." Certainly, steroids do have a very bad profile in the press. We know that long-term use of oral steroids can cause a great many serious health problems, and aerosols are not without their concerns. But we have also learned two important factors about steroids. One is that we know how to limit the impact on the rest of the body when the aerosol steroid stays in the airways. Secondly, we have learned the importance of using an anti-inflammatory medication. And, while I am loath to urge patients to use drugs that frighten them, aerosol steroids are often an essential part of treating this type of pulmonary disease. At its heart, obstructive pulmonary lung disease is an inflammatory process and, if we don't tackle this inflammation, we create two problems: (1) by treating just the symptoms, we can be masking a continuing underlying disease process that causes irreversible remodeling of the airways and lungs, and (2) this progressive damage from unchecked inflammation will require higher and higher doses of the bronchodilators and the other nonsteroidal antimediators. This will then increase the side effects to the point where they may be unbearable and even dangerous.

When a patient comes to me and doesn't want steroids, I will respect his or her anxiety about them and I will try alternatives. At the same time I will urge them to at least give the steroids a try. We don't want to see people lose pulmonary function, which is what happens if the inflammation continues unchecked.

Tailoring the Treatment

When people with COPD first come to me, they often have a bad cough that is actually an acute bronchitis. In this situation, I prescribe seven to ten days of antibiotics, in addition to bronchodilators. I like to use a long-acting bronchodilator to keep the patient feeling comfortable throughout the day and night. COPD is always there. Even if you respond well to the short-acting medication, after a few hours you will start to feel an increasing shortness of breath. You will need to reach for a short-acting inhaler, often at times that are not convenient. For example, patients who are teachers, lawyers, or performers can't just stop what they are doing and take a puff or two from an inhaler.

I often include a prescription for an inhaled steroid. The use of inhaled steroids in COPD has been controversial. Most doctors agree that 15–25 percent of people with COPD also have asthma and for them steroids definitely help reduce inflammation. I have found that many of my nonasthmatic COPD patients also do very well with inhaled steroids. They report less shortness of breath and seem to have fewer acute episodes. However, when acute exacerbations do occur, most doctors agree that steroids are necessary to control inflammation and symptoms and prevent accelerated damage to the lungs. In these cases, a short course of oral steroids may be necessary. Episodes of acute illness are a critical time when you have COPD. The inflammation in the airways in a full-blown infection can cause a sharp and permanent decline in lung function. I have had patients who were doing well until a bad respiratory infection destroyed so much lung tissue that they needed continual oxygen therapy when they left the hospital.

Depending on your symptoms, I will add a combination of short-acting beta agonists and anticholinergic bronchodilators. In some cases, low doses of theophylline can bring additional relief. I have found that my bigger and heavier patients can tolerate theophylline easier and report fewer side effects.

Combination therapy with different types of medications is the accepted standard for most people with chronic lung problems. Each one has a unique role in relieving symptoms and preventing further lung damage. Make it a priority to see that the prescriptions are not running out and that they are immediately accessible to you in your pocket or purse. Get into the "Sunday Night Survey" habit. Every Sunday evening, check that your medications are ready to go out with you on Monday morning. Check the dates on the prescriptions to make sure they are not empty or expired. If anything is needed, promise yourself the first stop the next morning is your drugstore.

When More Is Needed

Sister Mary Catherine has been my patient for more than fifteen years. Diagnosed with alpha-1 antitrypsin related emphysema when she was in her late forties, she liked to say that with her faith in God and my skill she felt her health was in good hands. But after three acute exacerbations that required hospitalization, Sister Mary Catherine found herself very short of breath. She could no longer teach math at the New York City parochial school where she had helped generations of girls master calculus and advanced algebra. In fact, even sitting quietly, she felt breathless. During a six-minute treadmill test, her O_2 saturation dipped into the low eighties, a clear sign that her lungs could not supply enough oxygen to meet her needs. Because medication could no longer improve her breathing, I knew it was time for supplemental oxygen therapy. I also knew that like most of my patients with COPD, Mary Catherine would resist the idea.

To ease her into the therapy, I suggested using oxygen while she slept at night. Eight hours of O_2 made her feel so much better, that she was able to resume at least part of her teaching schedule. Now comfortable with the idea of O_2 replacement therapy, she agreed to use O_2 in her office and when she was at home.

Studies have shown that O_2 improves strength and energy, reduces stress on the heart and even increases mental focus and concentration. Even more encouraging, using O_2 at least nineteen hours a day doubled survival rates over a twenty-six-month period. Ideally I would like to see my patients like Mary Catherine use oxygen at least eighteen hours a day, but I will always try to work out a compromise that both my patients and I can accept.

Different Forms of Oxygen

There are three types of O_2 delivery systems. *Compressed* oxygen is stored in a tank with a meter and regulator. This is a good choice if you are using oxygen just for several hours a day. This system can be made more efficient by using an oxygen conserving device that only releases the oxygen when you inhale. This prolongs the life of a portable tank and reduces its weight.

When O_2 is needed continuously I recommend *liquid oxygen*. This form comes in a large container that keeps the O_2 cold and liquid, allowing you to store large amounts at home. This form is probably the most suitable for portable oxygen. The oxygen can easily be transferred from the large reservoir to a small portable tank that weighs only a few pounds and can be carried in a sling like a purse allowing you to stay active. A conserving device can be used with this system.

An *oxygen concentrator* extracts oxygen from the air and delivers it through nasal prongs. Powered by electricity, the concentrator works beautifully for people who are not very active, but who need O_2 continuously. It is one of the most cost effective systems.

Private insurers, HMOs, as well as both Medicaid and Medicare, provide reimbursement for oxygen therapy as long as patients meet specific requirements. In his prescription for oxygen, a physician must give a diagnosis, results of lab tests that show blood saturation levels of less than 88 percent (or an equivalent blood gas result), and the amount of time O_2 therapy is needed each day, as well as the dose in liters per minute. In addition, the doctor usually has to specify therapeutic goals, such as improved ability to get around or to take care of oneself. Due to legislative changes to Medicare during 1998, reimbursement has been increasingly complex for patients to get complete coverage for the type and amount of O_2 they need. If you are experiencing problems with your health care insurers, ask your physician for help in untangling the red tape.

Lung Reduction Surgery

During a July heat wave for which New York City is justly famous, I got a call from a former medical student from Yale. Celeste, who was now a family physician in Westchester, asked me to see a fifty-year-old man with advanced COPD. Mr. Patel was taking the maximum levels of steroids and bronchodilators, and used O_2 supplementation at least twenty hours per day, but he still was very short of breath. Even simple daily tasks like eating a sandwich or taking a quick shower or shaving left him exhausted for hours. Celeste felt Mr. Patel was a good candidate for a somewhat controversial operation known as lung volume reduction surgery (LVRS) and she wanted my opinion on the best course to take.

LVRS removes up to 30 percent of diseased and damaged areas of one or both lungs. If you think back to Chapter Two, the tiny alveoli in the lungs become weakened, enlarged, and torn. By removing the most damaged, no longer functioning tissue, we allow the rest of the still functioning lung more room to expand. After surgery, pulmonary function tests show that the vital capacity or FEV1 may be significantly improved.

LVRS also improves the position of the diaphragm permitting a higher normal position that allows for easier breathing. The surgery even helps cardiac function because the operation has removed the overinflated tissue that was pressing on and blocking blood flow from returning to and exiting the heart. This situation can lead to a specific form of heart disease known as Cor Pulmonale.

When I examined Mr. Patel, I found that he was an excellent candidate for the surgery. Mr. Patel met all the current guidelines for this procedure. His FEV1 was 35 percent, he did not have severe heart disease and did not smoke cigarettes, abuse alcohol, or use drugs. During the five hour procedure, surgeons discovered a small, still localized lung cancer that had escaped detection with an X ray or even a CAT scan. We were able to remove it completely, preventing the spread of the lung cancer and its consequences.

Mr. Patel did well after the operation, and for two years, he felt like a new man. Not only could he enjoy daily life again, he went back to work and even traveled to visit his family in Bombay. But after several years, his lung function declined and he was again weak and breathless.

While LVRS can provide relief to a select group of patients, the benefits often do not last. In addition, clinical trials of the surgery indicate that LVRS does not increase survival time. Currently, there is an eighteen-center, five-year study that is following more than 2,000 patients with COPD. Directed by the National Heart, Lung, and Blood Institute, the study will measure and compare outcomes between LVRS and traditional treatments.

To date LVRS carries its own risks. Patients often have complications during and after surgery that include infections and strokes. Some patients die during or shortly after the procedure. Successful outcomes are often dependent on the skill and experience of the surgical team. If you are considering this operation, it is important to investigate the statistics of both the surgeon and his hospital. Ask the doctor how many LVRS procedures he has performed and what is their mortality rate. These are hard questions to ask, but you need to find the most competent and experienced people in your area for this serious decision.

Lung Transplantation

Replacing a diseased lung with a healthy one is arguably one of the most difficult types of transplant surgery, but for some patients it can offer a renewed sense of health and well-being. But before going into the operating room, there are a number of obstacles to overcome. Healthy lungs for transplant are very hard to come by. They are in such short supply that the surgeon will usually split a set of lungs between two patients. People are not put on the lung transplant list until they are given a prognosis of twelve to twenty-four months to live. Since most patients wait at least a year on the transplant list, it is often a race against time to find an appropriate donor. Too many people die before an organ becomes available for them.

To increase the odds of a positive outcome, surgeons follow strict patient selection guidelines. A good candidate needs to be under sixty-five, and does not smoke, use drugs, or abuse alcohol. In addition, the patient needs to be free of other chronic diseases such as diabetes, cancer, or liver failure.

Transplantation surgery does not end with the operation. The patient may need to take as many as sixty pills a day to prevent rejection of the new organ. They have to return every month for an invasive fiber optic procedure known as a bronchoscopy to see what bacteria are present in the airway and to spot signs of rejection.

In the short run, 65 percent of patients with COPD survive

the first year after surgery. But by the end of three years, only 20 percent of the people who have received a lung transplant will be alive. Clearly lung transplantation is not an easy choice to make, but for some patients who have no other options, it may provide years of active and productive life.

[Chapter 10]

The Healthy Home

T hroughout high school and college, Peter Kandinsky had been a star athlete. Just a few years after graduation, he had leveraged his talents and had become a very successful sports agent. In a single week, he could be found playing golf in Scotland, negotiating a burger endorsement for a basketball client in L.A., and cheering his pitcher at Yankee Stadium. Talented and energetic, he bought his first home at twenty-seven, a dream condo on Long Island. More than 2,000 square feet with great views of the sea, the condo complex included a golf course and tennis courts. To share in his good fortune, Peter invited his brother, Hank, who was a sophomore at a nearby college, to live with him. Less than three months after they moved in, the brothers noticed a foul odor from their basement. Engineers hired by the property managers reported that ground water had seeped into the basement of their home. They brought in sump pumps, resealed the walls, and assured the Kandinskys that their troubles were over. They were wrong.

Within a week, Peter and Hank began to cough and wheeze. They felt ill and exhausted and had to cut back on their schedules. Now Peter could barely get through the day and had to turn some of his top clients over to colleagues. Hank, who had also been on the football team, could no longer keep up. Even when they moved out of their condo, their health problems continued. An environmental consultant performed microbiological testing on the damaged house and found large quantities of mold living in the walls and in the floor spaces of the Kandinskys' home. Pulmonary function tests showed that these once exceptionally fit brothers had developed hyperactive airways from the mold that grew in their damp basement. Now living with their parents, they had to leave all their possessions behind because they were too contaminated with mold spores. Their recovery is very slow and it is likely that their health problems will persist for a long time to come.

It is hard to think of another condition where home design and care play a larger role in the maintenance of health than in chronic pulmonary disease. At home and in the workplace, there are allergens and irritants that can challenge sensitive airways. Fortunately, we are far from helpless. Through a number of practical strategies and accommodations, you can control both your environment and your health.

The Healthy Home

My patients are often concerned about industrial pollution, and in many cases, their concern is well founded. But they are less aware of the routine pollution issues in their own homes that are much more serious for their health. We spend up to 90 percent of our time indoors, and yet it is in the privacy and security of our home that you will find the most serious forms of pollution. The EPA estimates that the level of irritants are 5 to 100 times greater inside the home than outdoors.

From the basement to the attic, there are allergens and irritants that provoke symptoms and illness. In this chapter, I want to give you an overview of air quality issues in the home in general, and then, starting from the bottom to the top, I'm going to take you on a tour of your home. I will point out areas of potential problems and offer concrete and practical solutions. As we move along from room to room, keep in mind that you don't have to take action on every source of potential indoor air pollutant to improve air quality. I just want you to be aware of potential problems that may be at the root of your discomfort, not to frighten you into stripping your home of all furnishings.

Clearing the Air

The key to maintaining good air quality in the home depends on the right form of ventilation, which means balancing of the influx of outdoor air, which may carry pollen or by-products of car emissions, against the buildup of gases, allergens, and irritants that occur naturally in the home.

Old-style houses had plenty of ventilation. The wood and plaster construction was loose enough to allow sufficient air exchanges with the outside environment. But in the spaces and cracks in wood joints and masonry, you could develop excessive moisture, leading to mold and insect infestation. In addition, such houses were very expensive to heat. To make houses more energy-efficient, as well as to protect them from the outside pollution, we began to seal off our homes and offices. We increased insulation, added watertight weather seals to doors and windows, and even hung double-glazed glass at the windows. Our heating bills certainly went down, but the levels of indoor air pollutants soared. These types of hermetically sealed constructions led to the "sick building syndrome." Healthy people would develop symptoms such as chest tightness, headache, and coughing when they spent time inside such a building, and the symptoms would subside when they left.

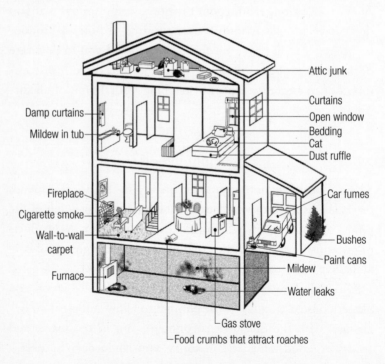

From the basement to the attic, air quality problems can develop in all areas of your home.

There were a lot of red faces several years ago when the new Environmental Protection Agency building in Washington turned out to have problems with indoor air pollution.

The new type of energy-efficient construction has made the houses warmer, but because they are warmer, they increased the amount of water condensation within the walls, leading to the growth of molds and to an accumulation of other organic materials. Although leaks from the ceilings or in the basements are less common, there is now an even more insidious type of moisture. It is the condensation of water between the cold outside walls and the warm interior which creates a hidden layer of humidity that can cause the growth of mold within the walls. The spores can then be released through the air vents and ceiling vents. You can't see the condensation or mold, but symptoms can definitely result from this pollution.

Caution: Fresh Air Can Be Hazardous to Your Health

On the other hand, if you leave your windows open for fresh air, you also can let in undesirable pollen, dust, and pollution from car exhaust and industry. In winter, cold dry air can provoke sensitive airways to narrow. I believe the right balance depends on a careful approach to ventilation. I would avoid sealing up the house too tightly. But at the same time, I recommend keeping windows protected most of the time. To eliminate dust and pollen, I would like to see you use "trickle ventilation" with adjustable window filters. They fit between the window and the windowsill, allowing entry of fresh air while trapping over 95 percent of the outdoor pollen. They do not stop gases such as ozone and NO_2, but are very helpful

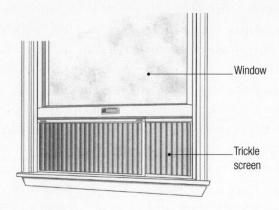

The trickle ventilation screen placed in an open window allows stale air to escape yet blocks dust, soot, and pollen from entering your home.

against plant allergens and particulate matter. When used in the kitchen, they allow you to clear the air of gas stove emissions and smoke, as well as cooking odors.

In spring and summer, I recommend running air-conditioning throughout the home. These machines "condition" the air in the room, removing moisture and venting it to the outside. Not only do they cool this air, many pollutants that dissolve in the moisture are also eliminated from your home. A good air conditioner will also remove large irritant particles, such as smoke and pollen.

For extra protection, add a high-performance micro particle filter such as Filtrete from 3M to your air conditioner. They can be cut to size to fit most makes and models of the air-conditioning unit. Use the old filter as a size guide and attach with masking tape. To keep an air conditioner running at peak efficiency, vacuum the coils every two weeks and change the filter every two to three months.

If you live in a single-family home, an attic fan that vents to the outside has been shown to lower pollutants in the rest of the house. It is an inexpensive way to add additional ventilation and improve indoor air quality.

All-Season Allergies

Although most pollen is usually a springtime issue, Christmas trees and foliage can be a problem for some people in the winter. In our apartment in New York City, a very charming Canadian couple comes down each December with a load of trees and sets them up outside our apartment building for sale. Unfortunately, my family is allergic to the oil in the evergreens and we have to keep our windows totally shut while the trees are piled up outside. If we try to open the window, several of us start to cough and sniffle almost immediately.

To improve indoor air quality, I recommend using a portable air-cleaning unit that contains a high-efficiency particulate air or HEPA filter. This powerful filter removes 95 percent of even the smallest particles suspended in the air and can remove larger particles such as pollen, dust mites, dog dander, and cat allergens. They are designed and priced for different-size rooms. Take care to choose the most efficient size for your room. The manufacturer will give you the dimensions of the room they can handle. Measure the size of your room, and if there is any doubt, choose the larger size. For example, suppose your room is 224 square feet. One model covers 168 square feet, the other covers 320 square feet. Although your room area falls between the two, select the larger filter to be sure that your air is as clean as possible.

These machines take about one hour to remove pollutants

from a room. In the bedroom, you should run them for about an hour before you go to sleep and then run it through the night. In living spaces, they can be used for several hours each day.

To provide maximum benefits, both air conditioners and HEPA air cleaners should be serviced regularly. If you have a central air-conditioning unit in your home, you should check the ducts once a month to remove any extra water that may have accumulated in them. HEPA filters tend to become clogged with pollen and dust and should be changed at least twice a season. HEPA air cleaners are rated on their ACH or air changes per hour. Each ACH represents circulating the volume in a room through the air cleaner one time. I recommend an ACH of six, that is to say, the cleaner provides six complete changes of air per hour.

There are other products offered for controlling air quality that are not nearly as effective as HEPA air cleaners or air-conditioning with micro particle filters. Ionizing air cleaners are designed to clean the air by ionizing particles in the air and having them settle on the walls and floors. This may work for a very short time, but activity and air currents in a room will stir them up and put them back into the air you breathe. In some of the older models, ionizers actually give off ozone, which is harmful, and I do not recommend them. Electronic filters charge particles of pollutants and deposit them on a filter. These tend to get filled very quickly, overloading their cleaning capacity. They need to be wiped clean almost daily, an activity that may send pollutants right back into your environment.

Humidifiers, which are designed to put moisture back into your home environment, can cause more problems than they solve. The moist warm environment of a humidifier offers a very hospitable environment for bacteria and molds. As you run the humidifier, you may be aerosolizing mold and bacteria. Even if you try to clean these machines very carefully, you may be aerosolizing the residue of cleaning fluid. Increasing the humidity in your home also makes it more comfortable for allergen-producing insects.

For maximum health and comfort, keep the relative humidity in your home between 40 and 50 percent. You can test the humidity with a simple combination thermometer/hygrometer available in most garden stores. If the humidity gets too low, it can be controlled by lowering your furnace or air-conditioning setting. Don't buy a humidifier, and if you own one, get rid of it.

A Healthy Heating, Ventilating, and Air-Conditioning (HVAC) System

The type and style of heating system in your home can play a large role in your pulmonary health. There are three types of heating systems, and each have benefits and drawbacks.

In the *Hot Water* or *Steam Heat System,* a home or apartment is heated by hot water circulated through pipes that run through the structure and is distributed by radiators or convectors. In a *Warm Air System,* air ducts circulate warmed air throughout the home. This forced air system uses a blower to push the air from the furnace in the basement up to the attic. The warm air travels through a series of ducts that enter a room via grills in the floor or walls.

Both hot water and warm air systems are powered by an oil-

or gas-run furnace and these fossil fuels give off emission pollutants. *Electrical Heating Systems,* which use radiant cables embedded in the ceilings or floors, do not give off pollutants and are recommended in homes designed for people with respiratory problems. Installed when a home is still under construction, they are economical to build but more expensive to run.

To improve the health profile of your existing heating system, take steps to modify and maintain your current machinery. Make certain that the furnace is vented outside your home. Replace the standard furnace filter (which is designed to keep the fan area clean) with a high-performance filter that captures small particulate matter before it can be blown into your home. Check with your heating company if your heating system can handle the additional filtration. In most forced-air systems, the filter is located close to the blower unit. There are over forty different sizes of high performance furnace filters such as Filtrete from 3M and you should be able to find one that fits the make and model of your heating system.

These filters pick up smoke, asbestos, and molds before they can be blown throughout your home. They are ranked by their MERV (minimum efficiency reporting value) rating, which measures the ability to trap particles in the air that are one micron or less. You want to look for a filter that can trap over 95 percent of the smallest particles. Manufacturers usually recommend changing the furnace filter every three months. If you live in an area with high dust levels due to dry weather, pollution, or construction, you may need to change the filter more frequently.

Attention also needs to be paid to the duct work in a forced-air heating system. Dirt, construction debris, and mold can accumulate in the maze of ducts that snake through the walls of your home. Keeping them clean and healthy is definitely not a do-it-yourself project. You need to hire a reputable duct-cleaning service. Never let them clean with chemicals, which can leave a residue that will be blown for months through your home.

In newer homes, central air-conditioning is often installed in the same ducts. Be sure to vacuum the air conditioner coils every three months and use a high-performance filter to pick up allergens and irritants. Keep in mind that a central heating, ventilation, and air-conditioning system (known as HVAC) can be modified with a central HEPA air-cleaning capability. However, this type of HEPA filter functions only when the heating or cooling units are operating. For complete protection, you may still need individual portable HEPA units, especially in the bedrooms.

A Costly Way to Save Money

To keep down heating costs, it may be tempting to use a space heater. Don't even think about it. These unvented kerosene or oil heaters emit fumes that will irritate your airways.

Wall Worries

Dust and chemicals also stick to walls and carpets from which they escape, slowly polluting the air in your home for long periods of time. The walls of your home can be an important source of air pollutants, particularly from paint or wallpaper. Wallpaper is a potent food for both dust mites and mold, which can grow behind the wallpaper. You will not see it, but your lungs will certainly know it is there.

I recommend using plain, flat, washable paint on all wall surfaces. Oil-based paints can be particularly irritating, and the odor can linger for some time. Latex paints dry quicker with less odor, but can still irritate highly sensitive people. If you have a significant problem with paint, I suggest resin-based paints. These specialty products do not contain the volatile compounds that are usually out-gased for months from the traditional wall paints. Low allergen paint, particularly on your bedroom walls, can be very helpful. See the Resources Section in the back of this book for stores that stock this product.

Put Your Airways on a Solid Footing

Flooring throughout the house is an important issue, and I strongly counsel my patients with lung problems to avoid wall-to-wall carpeting and to limit area rugs to the smallest possible size their decorating sense can tolerate. Carpets harbor everything you don't want to be breathing in. Pollen, dust, smoke, bacteria, and mold get buried in the carpet and are stirred up into the air when you walk on them. Even when brand-new, some carpet fibers can be irritating. Vacuuming, even daily, will not get all these pollutants and often just stirs them up.

I have had patients like Susan Schwartz, who would, each winter, develop a cold that would become bronchitis. From October to March, she would have repeated episodes of wheezing and coughing. When a pipe burst in her bathroom and caused a flood, she had to take up the sodden carpet in her bedroom. In the weeks that followed, she was amazed at the

difference in her health pattern. She was so pleased by her freedom from allergy and asthma symptoms that she took up the
carpeting in every room and replaced it with small area rugs
that she cleans every two to three months.

Try to keep carpeting out of your bedroom. If you have
pets, carpeting should be almost nonexistent throughout your
home. You cannot get the traces of pet saliva and urine out of a
carpet. Molecules of these allergens will be stirred up each time
you walk on the carpet and hang in the air for hours. I like to
see my patients be on the least possible medication with the
best possible symptom control, and I have found that removing
carpeting can have more impact on pulmonary health than a
row of new medications.

Pets are a different story. While there may be some attachment to new carpeting or comfortable bedding, the emotional
link to pets is on an altogether different level of magnitude.
The direct approach usually has little chance of being successful. On the other hand, an indirect approach may help con-
vince some. I frequently will ask if the pet can be boarded at
some family or friend's house for a short period of time, two to
four weeks. If this results in a significant reduction of symptoms, this short separation may be a way to explore other
options.

A Lung's Tour of Your Home Environment

The respiratory-friendly home starts outside with the control
of pollen and mold on your property. Pollens are minute oval
male cells found in many plants. Those with bright flowers like
roses have larger, heavier pollen grains that are carried from

plant to plant by bees and insects. Grasses and trees have very small pollen grains that are transmitted by the wind. In the spring, pollens from oak, cedar, elm, and maple trees are common causes of allergy symptoms. In the summer, grasses provoke allergies and asthma. From late summer to early fall, weeds like ragweed and thistle cause problems. Flowers related to ragweed, including mums, zinnias, and dahlias, which bloom at this time, can be equally troublesome. It is estimated that in the United States and Canada, over 300 million tons of pollen are circulated in August and September.

Do Pollen Counts Count?

The National Allergy Bureau compiles pollen counts of trees, weeds, and grasses throughout the United States and issues the findings three times a week. Season, weather, and sampling techniques will affect measurements. Many people react when pollen counts are in the moderate range, but reactions are very individual. In general, allergists suggest that sensitive people stay indoors and keep their air conditioners running when pollen counts are categorized as high.

To keep pollen levels low on your property, keep shrubs and trees at least three feet away from your home. If allergy seems to play a large role in your breathing problems, consider replacing pollen-rich grass with a low ground cover, such as vincor minor. In your garden, avoid landscaping fragrant or flowering plants. In the autumn, pick up fallen leaves before they become wet and matted. Spring cleaning should include removal of fallen branches, leaves, and patches of moss. Never spray insecticides or weed killers to control the landscaping.

These poisonous compounds are also highly irritating to even healthy airways. Finally, two to four times a year, clear gutters and drain pipes before trapped leaves can decay and mold.

Cleaning Out the Garage

No matter how hard we try, the garage tends to become the dumping ground for the rest of the house. It's not the clutter that concerns me, but the fumes from a number of different sources that accumulate there. If you have an attached garage, the fumes from your car can seep into your house. To avoid breathing in your own homemade carbon monoxide and dust particles, make certain that the doors between the garage and your home are always shut. These doors are a good place to install weather stripping to prevent seepage. It can also be very helpful to install an exhaust fan in the garage that is set to run for fifteen minutes each time you drive in and out.

Your car isn't the only problem in the garage. This is also an area where you store paint cans, fertilizers, strong cleaning supplies, and insecticides, all of which give off volatile compounds. Make sure they are tightly closed and keep them far away from the door between your home and the garage.

Getting to the Bottom of Your Pulmonary Problems

Some of the most stubborn air quality problems start in your basement, where damp cold air is an open invitation to heavy mold growth. Mold is a form of fungus that thrives in warm, moist environments. The most common form of household mold is black mildew, which also makes an appearance upstairs in bathroom grout tiles and on shower curtains. Problems arise when the molds release spores into the air. When inhaled, these spores settle in the airways, where they cause inflammation and irritation in sensitive lungs. In the basement, the close proximity to the ground also promotes an accumulation of dust and dirt. Even if you never set foot in your basement, mold spores and dust make their way through the cracks in your floor and through heating vents into the living areas above.

You can start controlling your basement environment by controlling the humidity. Hang a combination humidity/temperature gauge in the basement to measure the level of moisture. To discourage the growth of mold and bacteria, you want to keep humidity levels between 40 and 50 percent. If humidity levels are consistently higher, look for sources of moisture. Some sources of moisture are easy to spot, such as a leaky washing machine, or a loose fitting on a water pipe. Check the basement while it's raining to spot cracks and leaks in the walls that are a source of water infiltration. Once identified, these can be caulked and sealed.

One of the best ways to control basement moisture is to buy a portable dehumidifier. Be sure to have the dehumidifier vent to the outside, or regularly empty the bucket to prevent the accumulation of water. If you have a washing machine and dryer in your basement, make sure that the dryer is vented to the outside to avoid spraying fine airborne particles of fiber into the house, as well as an aerosol of moisture condensation.

The basement is also the site of most home-heating units. In general, any home-heating system that uses fuel (i.e., oil or gas), produces by-products that can trigger respiratory problems. In addition to using a high-performance or micro particle filter in a blower system, environmental experts suggest enclosing the furnace in a small room within the basement to contain the by-products of combustion that could escape from the pipes and vents. You may also find that the pipes have been wrapped with asbestos insulation material. If it is old and cracked, hire experts to remove it. Never try to deal with asbestos yourself. You can injure your lungs, as well as spread asbestos fibers throughout your home.

A Living, Breathing Room

Moving upstairs to the living room, we need to look at the furniture. My first concern with furniture is the type of wood. Many types of moderately priced, modern furniture use particle board or pressed wood that is made of slivers of wood bound together with adhesives made with large amounts of chemicals called isocyanates. These isocyanates act as a binding agent, causing particles to stick together, as in paints or in pressed wood. When these items are new, the outgassing of these chemicals can be a significant trigger for asthma or lung irritation. If you are looking for new furniture, I would avoid this type entirely. If you have older furniture made with these chemicals, much of the irritating gases may have already been dissipated to the air. If you are in the market for furniture, my first choice would be modern pieces constructed of solid wood. They are more expensive, but may reduce medical bills and sick days.

Older pieces, such as golden oak or country pine, are solid wood but depending on where they've been stored and aged, they also can be sources for mold. To remove any mold from vintage furniture, sponge it down with a dilute solution of bleach. Don't forget to sponge down the drawers and the back area, which is where the mold commonly accumulates. Let the smell of the bleach evaporate into the air before bringing the furniture into your home. It is only necessary to do this when you bring an antique find home for the first time. Once housed in a heated, controlled environment of a home, mold will no longer develop.

Healthy Decorating

In an ideal pulmonary environment, there would be relatively few objects to catch dust, but few of us want to live in that sterile an environment. We all have books and mementos that we love to see around us. Unfortunately, they are allergen magnets that constantly release their molecules into the air. If your respiratory symptoms are severe, you can try enclosing your books and your decorative pieces behind glass to avoid dust accumulation. On shelves and tables, books should be wiped down with an electrostatic cloth at least every two weeks to eliminate buildup of dust and pollen particles.

Vacuum your soft upholstery furniture, like couches and sofas, once a week to remove loose dust, pollen, and mites that can accumulate there. Some doctors suggest using only vinyl or leather furniture. But, unless the symptoms require it, I don't recommend it for the majority of my patients. Routine cleaning with a hardy vacuum cleaner will eliminate many of these allergens.

The safest and most effective vacuum cleaners use a HEPA filter, like the ones recommended for cleaning the air. These are more expensive, but studies have shown that they do pick up an enormous amount of these pollutants and they don't spread them around in the air during cleaning. There are also HEPA vacuum cleaners or attachments that work effectively on hardwood floors and pick up almost all traces of dirt and dust.

While you are in a cleaning mode, keep in mind that electrostatic cloths and wipes such as Swiffer also do an excellent job of picking up loose dust, pollen, and particulates without spreading them around the room, as you would with a broom or feather duster.

Detailed carving on picture frames, decorative items, or furniture catch dust and can be the source of irritants as these particles become airborne again. These items should be cleansed with electrostatic wipes every week. It can be very helpful to clean off the glass-framed pictures on the walls once a week, making sure that the top of the picture frame is dusted. This is where a great deal of pollutants accumulate and are reaerosolized when people move around a room. When shopping for new home furnishings, especially for the bedroom, look for the straightest, simplest lines and avoid adding new dust catchers.

If you suffer from respiratory problems, be very careful not to provoke more problems for yourself as you clean your home. By wearing glasses or goggles and a HEPA filter mask that fits tightly on your face around the nose and mouth, you can avoid breathing in these pollutants as you dust or vacuum. If you find that cleaning brings on wheezing, have someone else do these chores and stay out of the home while cleaning is actually occurring.

Don't dust or vacuum a room less than three hours before you go to sleep. Cleaning will stir up dust and irritants that can irritate sensitive airways at night. To prevent problems, do your housework in the morning to allow allergens to settle down.

Private Spaces: The Bedroom

It is no coincidence that many of the most serious asthma attacks occur at night, since one of the most powerful asthma-provoking allergens hides in your bedroom. Each night you inhale large amounts of allergens produced by dust mites. These are microscopic creatures that are related to ticks and spiders, but, unlike their more aggressive cousins, they do not sting or spread disease. They are happy to live quietly on dust, mold, and pollen and especially love the dead skin cells that we shed each day. Unfortunately, their droppings are a major cause of allergic asthma. It is estimated that the average bed contains more than 10,000 dust mites and greater than 2 million droppings. Dust mites are incredibly hard and tenacious. They burrow deep into carpets, bedding, and upholsteries. Their highly irritating droppings are so tiny that when stirred up by the presence of people in a room, they can remain airborne for thirty minutes before settling back on beds, carpets, and other softer furniture. Controlling dust mites, particularly in the bedroom, is an important goal for the relief of asthma and allergic diseases.

Dust mites flourish in warm, moist environments. By keeping room temperature below seventy-seven degrees, you will discourage their growth. Moisture is usually not an issue in the bedroom, but dust accumulation, which feeds the mites in and around your bed, is a frequent problem. To keep down levels of dust mite allergens, avoid dust ruffles, try not to store anything under beds, and vacuum the bedroom (particularly under the beds) several times a week. Dust mites are particularly happy with pile carpets, which is why I urge my patients to keep their bedrooms free of floor coverings.

Changing bed linen once a week is helpful, but dust mites tend to burrow deep into mattresses and cannot even be dislodged with a thorough vacuuming. To protect your bedding, I recommend encasing both your mattress and pillows in antimite barrier covers. These items prevent contact with dust mites in your bedding. New mites may appear on this cover, but will be dislodged when you change your sheets. To take extra precautions, wipe the surface of the barrier cover with a slightly damp cloth to remove mites and skin scales. Once made of stiff, uncomfortable plastic, antimite covers are now formed of soft, clothlike material. They should be machine-washed in very hot water twice a year. Depending on the price and quality, these covers last from two to ten years. Avoid the use of down pillows and comforters, which can be themselves highly allergenic and are a favorite food of dust mites.

Dust mites are also the reason I recommend using shades or washable curtains, rather than drapes or complicated window treatments in the bedroom. Dust mites love to accumulate in padded headboards, canopies, and bed hangings. I would also suggest reducing clutter on your bedside tables and on your dresser, which can accumulate dust and dust mites. Finally, your bedspread, quilts, and blankets should also be washed frequently to reduce dust mite buildup. Epidemiological studies have shown that up to 70 percent of people with asthma are sensitive to dust mites, and controlling dust mites is a critical step in controlling pulmonary comfort.

There are antidust mite chemicals available but I would prefer not to add extra chemicals into your environment, especially where you sleep. I think that frequent vacuuming, a HEPA air filter, and carpet-free bedrooms will lower the dust mite load enough to avoid needing any other remedies that could introduce new problems.

Health Hazards of Dry Cleaning

When you take your clothes home from the dry cleaners, let them air out for a day to get rid of cleaning chemicals that can be irritating to your airways.

The Heart of the Home—The Kitchen

Whether it's big or small, the kitchen is the source of comfort and food for the whole family. The first issue that you should address in this room is the heat source of your stove and oven. Gas stoves, which I know are favored by the best cooks because they can control the heat, use a fossil fuel that creates nitrogen dioxide, a known pulmonary irritant. If you have a choice of a cooking stove, I would urge you to use electrical models. If that's not possible, be careful to have good ventilation when using your stove or oven. A hood that vents the air from the kitchen to the outside is a valuable tool for controlling emissions—one that simply recirculates the air does not help. Alternatively, I would urge you to keep a window open in the kitchen when you cook to encourage the elimination of these gases. If you have a galley kitchen in an apartment, then I would keep a window open in the nearest room while you are cooking.

The second issue in a kitchen is far less glamorous than gour-met cooking—cockroaches. These ubiquitous insects love food and water, and where will they find more of it but in a kitchen? Unlike dust mites, cockroaches are all too visible. Not only do they carry disease, they are highly allergenic, provoking severe asthmatic symptoms.

Researchers believe that it is the digestive enzyme in the roach droppings that provokes bronchoconstriction. Keeping the kitchen free of crumbs and mopping up water will discourage their invasion. Vacuuming the floor regularly will pick up traces of both food, as well as allergen-loaded roach droppings. If roaches are a problem, use roach traps along the baseboards under the sinks and in the corners of the bathroom. Avoid traditional insect sprays, which are extremely irritating to sensitive airways. Because roaches love water, make sure that you turn off your faucets tightly and that there are no leaks. Once a month, clean under your sink, mopping up any spots of water or dirt and checking for roach infestation.

When cleaning the kitchen, use disposable paper towels, rather than sponges, which can develop mold. Pick cleaning aids carefully. Look for fragrance formulas based on natural soaps and oil. Some of the least allergenic can be found in health food stores. Whatever you buy, avoid using pump or aerosol sprays because you don't want to add any chemicals into the air.

Inner Sanctums: The Bathroom

Compared to the bedroom, your bathroom has fewer places for allergens to lurk. These rooms rarely have wall-to-wall car-

peting, and those carpets that do exist are usually washed frequently. There are very few soft furnishings for dust mites to
burrow in. However, the high-moisture levels in the bath-
rooms are a source of serious mold development and can attract cockroaches.

To avoid moisture buildup, leave a window open a crack
while the bathroom is in use or use a small portable fan to dis-
perse the moisture. Be sure to throw away any plastic shower
curtains that show signs of mold and replace them with new
mold-resistant shower curtains. If possible, use roll-up shades or
frosted glass for privacy, rather than curtains. Even washable
curtains harbor mold, since the high moisture in a bathroom
will just keep them slightly damp all the time. If you have
shower doors, use a toothbrush to get into the narrow tracks,
in order to clean out all traces of mold that can accumulate.
When ventilation is a problem, use paper towels to wipe down
the tile walls after showers or baths to eliminate the moisture.
Make sure that you ventilate your bath mat after each use so
that it doesn't stay damp.

If mold does appear, it can be treated with dilute solutions of
bleach. Because bleach is irritating, have this done by someone
else or wear a mask and goggles if you are going to clean the
bathroom yourself. Don't use room fresheners, potpourri, or
aromatherapy candles, because these actually will aerosolize
fragrance irritants, and you're exchanging one problem for
another.

The Home Office

In the home office, the biggest problem is clutter. There has to be someplace in the home where you can put the papers and files that you need. Unfortunately, these can be a major source of dust mites, dust, and pollen. There can also be a release of ozone from electrical equipment, such as laser printers and photocopiers. To keep these pollutants low, offices should have bare floors and a minimum of decorative material. Try to keep papers in boxes, file cabinets, or stored behind glass to avoid the accumulation of dust. Go through your files every six months to eliminate anything that you just don't need. Plastic or stainless-steel trash cans are preferable to rattan or woven ones, which catch dust.

The Nondusty Attic

Almost by definition, attics are dusty, musty, and cluttered. But if you have irritable airways, traditional attic jumble can trigger problems in the rest of the house. On a rainy day, go into your attic and scan the ceilings for signs of moisture. A leaky roof will admit water into your home, undermining its structure and leading to the hidden and dangerous growth of mold. The attic leaks can also soak papers and clothing stored in the attic, promoting mold and mildew. To avoid increasing indoor air pollution, store unused items in clear plastic boxes. Repair leaks in the roof to reduce moisture accumulation, and vacuum every two months to capture pollen, dust mite allergens, and dirt particles. An exhaust fan vented to the outside can control heat, moisture, and accumulation of particulate matter.

Cleaning Strategies

Keeping dust and pollen levels down with daily cleaning is invaluable for improving indoor air quality, but it is important to avoid irritating cleansing products. Start by eliminating anything in a spray, both in pump and aerosol. Look for unscented products, and if these still provoke problems, use a tightly fitting HEPA mask when applying it. If you still develop chest tightness or shortness of breath, have someone else do the cleaning and leave the apartment or home while it's being done.

Most cleaning products contain chlorine, phosphates, or ammonia, all of which are irritating. But we still need these antibacterial and antifungal agents to do a thorough job. By eliminating the scents, we eliminate unnecessary irritants.

You can look in health food stores for ecologically safe products. It may not mean they are less irritating to a hair-trigger pulmonary system, but they generally are fragrance-free and have lower levels of volatile organic compounds, so they are usually better tolerated.

Using a strong vacuum cleaner equipped with a HEPA filter several times a week is invaluable for improving indoor air quality and is absolutely essential if there is a smoker or pets in the home. The vacuum cleaner should be examined monthly to make sure that it's functioning properly and that the bags need to be emptied. You should not use any cleaning product that moves dust around, such as a feather duster, dusting rag, or broom.

Electrostatic cloths, such as Swiffer, will pick up the dust as you move the cloth along it and tend not to send it airborne.

Use these cloths to pick up allergens on furniture and picture frames. Attached to a floor sweeper, electrostatic cloths pick up and remove dust, pollen, and pet dander. By contrast, sweeping with a broom can stir up allergens and provoke problems. Avoiding exposure to mold spores, dust mites, and dust allergens with good ventilation and cleaning techniques will dramatically reduce exposure to these pulmonary triggers.

"I Bet You Even Hate Lassie"

Discussing the link between asthma and the family pet is one of the most sensitive issues that comes up between me and my patients. The bond between a dog or cat and a patient can be as strong as between parent and child. Yet, when I have a patient like Sam Morris, I feel compelled to force a patient to make difficult choices. Sam had asthma, emphysema, and a pair of cocker spaniels that he adored. Unfortunately, his allergy to dog dander made it impossible to control his asthma. After his third visit to the emergency room in three months, I sat him down for a serious man/dog discussion. He listened silently as I explained the problems of dog allergy and his deteriorating lung condition.

When I finished, he looked at me sadly. "I bet you'd even ban Lassie," he said. Since Sam also smoked, we came up with a compromise. Either the cigarettes or the dogs had to go. The dogs stayed, and while Sam still has problems, those midnight runs to the emergency room have ceased.

Allergens found in pet hair, saliva, and urine are easily transferred to furniture and can hang in the air for hours. Cats seem to cause the greatest problems, with up to 40 percent of asthmatics showing some degree of sensitivity to felines. Dogs affect fewer people, but are still a problem for many with pulmonary sensitivity. The best options would be a pet-free home, but that is just not an acceptable option for many of my patients. To reduce problems, there are a number of strategies that can lower exposure.

The first rule is nonnegotiable: No pets in your bedroom. Keeping them out of the sleeping area, especially off the bed, has been shown to be effective for reducing symptoms of wheezing and congestion.

Bathing pets weekly at a professional facility is also very helpful, albeit an expensive strategy. Do not try to bathe pets yourself. If you are sensitive, the direct and intense exposure to the allergens can trigger an attack. Even if done by others in the home, the fuss and activity of bathing a usually not too eager pet will spread allergens throughout the air.

The presence of pets in the home make the use of portable HEPA air filters in both bedrooms and living areas a necessity, not an option. Floors should be cleaned with a high-performance vacuum cleaner equipped with a HEPA filter and it goes without saying that if you want your pet, you have to get rid of your wall-to-wall carpets. Better still, even avoid area rugs. These strategies do take extra time and money, but are very necessary if your pets and you are to live together safely and happily.

Pet allergies are not limited to dogs and cats. I recently had a patient whose granddaughter was given a pair of guinea pigs. Not only did she seem to develop asthmatic wheezing but also she actually had a full-blown anaphylactic reaction. These life-threatening responses to allergens can be characterized by chest tightness, body swelling, swelling inside the voice box, shock, and even death.

She wanted to see her granddaughter and didn't want to ask her to give up the pets. Even when the granddaughter came to visit her, the dander and hairs seemed to accompany the child who loved and played with her guinea pigs frequently. We looked into desensitizing her with allergy shots, but the allergists were uncomfortable with the idea and felt that success was far from guaranteed. So we prescribed an increased dosage bronchodilator and antihistamines to use when she saw her granddaughter. And it proved once again that there is no greater love than of a grandmother for her grandchild.

Tips for Apartment Dwellers

When you have asthma/COPD, there are benefits and challenges to living in an apartment. You will not have to worry about moldy leaves, grass pollen, and garage fumes. On the other hand, allergens from dust mites and roaches are major urban allergens. Emission from traffic and power plants can raise air pollution levels, particularly in warm weather areas. You also have no control of the condition of the heating system in your building. To improve indoor air quality, you will need to rely on high-performance HEPA filters in your vacuum cleaner, air conditioner, and portable room cleaners. Use "trickle ventilation" to keep out dust, pollen, and soot, yet allow gases and moisture to escape (see page 217).

Be careful with plants and flowers. Mold can develop on the soil of house plants, and the spores can induce an allergic response. As they age, cut flowers can shed their pollen, which will become airborne as you move around. Decorative objects, books, and clothing can accumulate large amounts of dust in the city. Keep clothing in drawers and closets and don't let piles of papers and magazines accumulate.

Use a fresh electrostatic cloth to wipe down framed pictures and tabletop collections. Regularly vacuum floors, bookshelves, under beds and radiators, and along the windowsills. I have found that a handheld HEPA vacuum gets into small nooks and tight spaces that harbor big sources of allergens and triggers in city apartments.

Outdoor Pollution—Natural and Unnatural

In summer months, patients who are sensitive to grasses and pollen will begin showing more symptoms, even if they live in a city environment. Pollen deposits itself in your hair, and when you go to sleep at night, the pollen is transferred to your pillow. By putting your face into the pillow, literally, you are directly inhaling pollen right down into the smallest airways of your lungs.

To reduce this pollen load, I recommend a shampoo and shower before going to bed. This has the dramatic effect of lowering the pollen load and preventing its transfer to bed linens. The warm sunny weather is not the only time when irritations to the lungs occur. That cold dry weather is a very well-known and a very common trigger for pulmonary distress. During the winter, many patients ask me if they should use a mask. I find that simply wrapping a scarf around your mouth and nose warms the air sufficiently to avoid bronchospasms.

Controlling the indoor environment can provide important pulmonary protection. If asthma is a problem, the reduction of irritants can decrease risk of wheezing and incidence of acute attacks. When chronic bronchitis and emphysema are causing symptoms, lower irritant levels can reduce risk of damaging inflammation.

Chapter 11

Healthy Lungs at Work and at Play

The potential health problems of the workplace are often very obvious. Workers in so-called dirty jobs, such as coal mining, steel, and cotton mills, have been routinely exposed to high levels of pollution that can lead to lung disease. In fact, many of these industries have their own distinct respiratory syndromes, such as black lung, seen in coal miners, and brown lung, also known as byssinosis, in cotton textile workers. The struggle to clean up these workplace environments has been going on for almost as long as there has been a workplace.

Occupational airway disease is not uncommon in a broad range of industries. For example, about 10 percent of workers exposed to isocyanates, a chemical used in spray paints, insulating materials, and foam, are reported to develop asthma. Up to 25 percent of people exposed to the enzymes used in the manufacture of detergents develop pulmonary problems. In the printing industry, up to 50 percent of employees develop wheezing or shortness of breath from constant exposure to gum acacia. This chemical is essential for color printing to separate sheets and for preventing the blurring of an image.

State-of-the-art ventilation and filtration is important to reduce the incidence of symptoms in these high-risk industries. Often, symptoms may be controlled with medication, but frequently it is best to move to another job with less exposure to irritants.

In recent years, the new and stronger regulations developed and enforced by OSHA (Occupational Safety and Health Administration) have made the workplace safer for the average worker. But occupational health problems exist, even in the seemingly cleanest environments, such as offices, schools, and hospitals. For people without risk of pulmonary disease, such environments usually do not pose difficulties, but for those with asthma, COPD, or simply for people who are smokers, breathing problems can be just around the corner.

Sick Building Syndrome

Office air pollution is so widespread that the Environmental Protection Agency (EPA) ranks indoor air quality among the top five environmental risks to public health. Often called "sick building syndrome" (SBS), it is characterized by symptoms such as headache, teary eyes, and sinus congestion. These nonspecific signs may affect a large number of usually healthy workers. For people with underlying respiratory problems, the environment in a sick building can produce long-term—and serious—health issues. Problems often arise when a new building is occupied before it has had time to air out gases and fumes produced by new construction materials or from an environmental disaster like that which affected my patients Peter and Hank Kandinsky in their condo. In addition, older buildings undergoing plastering, painting, and carpeting are also common factors in SBS. Each year I see several patients whose symptoms started when they continued to live or work in a building while renovations were under way.

What You Can Do

It can be much harder to exert control over your workplace air quality than your home, but changes can be made to reduce symptoms. Most buildings have a central heating, ventilation, and air-conditioning system known as HVAC. The air quality that they produce depends a great deal on the type of system, its efficiency, age, and maintenance schedule. If the windows cannot be opened in the building, the air quality and design is completely dependent on the design of this equipment—and minor problems in function can produce major problems in health. For example, mold growth from water accumulating in the duct system can be aerosolized throughout the building. Poorly maintained HVAC systems can also spray pollen and particulate matter into the office environment. Even when the system is in good working order, the levels of pollution in a tightly shut building can be more than a normal HVAC filtration unit can handle. If you are having a problem, check with your office manager to make sure equipment is being properly maintained.

Flooring is often a major source of problems in an otherwise clean workplace. Carpets harbor a constant source of allergen, mold, dust, and dust mites. The heavy flow of traffic through an office every day means that these allergens and irritants are

stirred up continuously and hang in the air. Even daily vacuuming can't control the level of allergens that build up in this
carpeting. Keeping a small HEPA filter in your work area or
on your desk can improve your air quality. Patients report that
it can make a remarkable difference in the way they feel.

Hardwood floors are much cleaner than carpets but, when
newly refinished, can off-gas or release volatile compounds that
can be irritating. This is usually a time-limited problem,
whereas carpeting is a long-term situation that only gets worse.
We certainly can't ask that a large company tear up the carpeting in their entire building, but you can keep a small HEPA
vacuum cleaner in your office to run over the carpet in your
personal space. A quick pass in the morning and in the evening
will keep the environment in your office as clean as possible.

Paper is also a source of compounds that can be irritating,
and there are infinite amounts of paper in every office. The
best way to deal with the off-gassing from chemical-rich paper
is to keep paper to a minimum and store it in files, cabinets, and
drawers, and not on the surface of your desk. You should try to
keep a minimum of items on the desk and a minimum of decorative items around your office, all of which are just ways to
catch additional dust and allergens.

Office furniture itself can be a problem, since it is often
made of less expensive particle board that contains large
amounts of formaldehyde. When new, this type of furniture
can off-gas volatile compounds. If you develop symptoms after
new furniture is installed in your office, this furniture might be
the source of your problems. You can apply special clear
sealants on the surface of your furniture to reduce the release of
irritating fumes into your air.

Avoid keeping a laser printer for your computer in your

office, since this is a source of ozone gas, which can upset hyperactive airways.

Although some people have suggested keeping plants in the offices as a source of oxygen, I have found that they can be a source of mold, whose spores become airborne and cause irritation.

For some patients, I've recommended that they shower and wash their hair after a day at the office before going to sleep. This will reduce the allergens that can have settled on their body. These allergens can be easily transferred to bed linens, where they can be inhaled all night.

You might think that the people who work in heavy industries have a higher incidence in asthma and allergies than those in office jobs, but actually what we usually find is what's called the "healthy worker effect." People with respiratory problems generally avoid working in polluted environments like steel mills or coal mines. If there is an underlying sensitivity to these irritants, people just simply cannot make any kind of long-term career in such a workplace. What we do see is the gradual development of new chronic lung diseases in people employed in a dusty workplace.

We have also found that there is a very troubling synergy between a contaminated workplace and cigarette smoking. For example, smokers who work in a coal mine or cotton mills have much higher rates and more severe forms of lung problems than do nonsmokers in the same situation.

I have seen firsthand the interaction of smoking and workplace contaminants. When I was at Yale, my family and I had just bought a turn-of-the-century house in New Haven that turned out to need a great deal of work. We had to hire people to repair and paint practically every room. At one point, we decided to restore the first floor to its former beauty. I hired a painter who was a superb craftsman and a man who really loved his job. He actually specialized in painting churches and he had some free time and was available to paint our rather elaborately plastered dining room and living room.

Al Lebow was a charming man of about sixty. A heavy smoker who had already had one heart attack, Al knew more about paint and color than anyone I had ever met. He was always in good spirits but often extremely short of breath. Yet, every few hours, he would step outside for a cigarette. When I offered to help him quit smoking, Al explained that painters needed to smoke to deal with the smells of his job. Shortly after finishing our house, Al underwent triple bypass surgery and was forced to retire.

Several months later, I looked up to find that the ceiling of my study had started to sag toward the floor. It looked like the entire ceiling was ready to collapse. Through Al, we found Joe Savinelli, "the man that taught me everything I knew about paint," Al assured me in a hoarse voice.

At eighty, Joe Savinelli walked with the snap and vigor of a man half his age. I watched in amazement as Joe nimbly climbed a ladder, poked a pin in my ceiling, and chuckled as a stream of powder poured down much the way sand comes through an egg timer. Sam had seen houses like mine when they both were young. He explained that in old Victorian-style homes, the ceilings were plastered and then—to keep the plaster in place—a piece of canvas was wet-glued to the surface. But over the last 100 years, the plaster had dried out, powdered, and now was pushing the canvas back down to the floor.

He told me he was going to take off the canvas and replaster the ceiling. I watched, fascinated, for the next few days as Joe worked much like Michelangelo when he worked on the ceiling of the Sistine Chapel. With his hands over his head for hours at a time, he removed the canvas and then replastered the ceiling. Remember, as we grow older, we lose lung function and use the muscles of the neck and shoulders to help us breathe. As a result, at his age, it should be more difficult to use these muscles for activities such as above-the-shoulder plastering and painting. Watching Joe work, it was clear that the physiology of aging didn't interest him.

Unlike Al, Joe never took a cigarette break and, as it turned out, "never got that dirty habit." Joe was still working when I left New Haven several years later. I never forgot the contrast between the health of the two at work in the same paint and plaster environment. Al, who smoked, had to retire in ill health twenty years before Joe, who continued working at a job he loved well into his eighties.

The Artist at Work

Watching Joe and Al sparked a continuing interest in the health problems of people who work with paints and other art material. Toxic exposure to art materials has been shown to affect painters, sculptors, photographers, and jewelry makers. They routinely breathe in unhealthy levels of asbestos, benzene, lead, acetates, and formaldehyde. Pigments, solvents, dyes, and metals are linked to a wide range of health concerns. These same chemicals are used in crafts and do-it-yourself projects, and can cause the same respiratory problems that I see in painters and other artisans in my practice.

The key to trouble-free art lies in adequate ventilation. Work in a large, well-aired place, run your HEPA filter as you work, and keep it running for two hours after you stop. Face masks are not of much help unless they are tight-fitting and are equipped with HEPA filters or are self-enclosed with an outside source of oxygen. If you tend to experience chest tightness or coughing, and have been prescribed a preventative bronchodilator, even with adequate ventilation, try taking a dose of short-acting bronchodilator shortly before beginning the arts and crafts activity.

Applying for Work-Related Disability

Jackson Brown had been a happy man. A deacon in his church and married for thirty years to his high school sweetheart, Mr. Brown ran his department with a firm but fair hand. It is hard to think of a cleaner and safer environment than the quiet university library where he worked, but it turned out to be the cause of his asthma. Mr. Brown had managed the maintenance department of the university library for fifteen years, when he began to cough and feel short of breath. The symptoms would get worse as the day went on and, often by the end of the week, he could barely walk. On the weekends, he would start to feel better, but once he was back to work, his problems would return. He soon used up his sick days and vacation time when he felt too ill to go to work. By the time I saw him, Mr. Brown was afraid he was going to lose his job.

In the course of his chest workup, it became apparent that he had recurrent episodes of bronchitis over the years, but he had just shrugged them off and continued to work. Lung function tests showed a decline in FEV1 and clear evidence of chronic bronchospasm. Because I felt that Mr. Brown's severe health problems were due to his long exposure to cleaning solutions, I suggested that he apply for Workman's Compensation.

The Right to a Safe Work Environment

Before the 1920s, a worker had to take an employer to court if he felt he had been injured on the job. This was an expensive and lengthy process, and most workers could not afford to pursue compensation. Since both time and the law were on the side of the employers, even if a worker tried to take the company to court, the bar was raised too high to prove the case.

Following World War I, Congress enacted the first of a number of no-fault laws designed to give workers the financial and medical support they needed and deserved. Today there are three major programs to help disabled employees: Workman's Compensation, Social Security Disability Insurance (SSDI), and Supplemental Security Income (SSI). These programs share two basic requirements:

- A diagnosis of a specific medical or psychological condition
- Proof that the condition makes it impossible to work at the job

Clearly, Mr. Brown satisfied both requirements. His symptoms and lung function tests showed that he had severe, persistent asthma; the health problems were acute at work and improved during the weekend; he had used up all his sick days and was in danger of losing his job.

Different Rates in Different States

Each state has its own version of Workman's Compensation. But the common feature is that the injury claimed is determined to be work-related. As a no-fault system, neither the worker nor the employer is to blame for the injury. In the past, employers would try to escape liability by claiming that a worker was careless, drunk, or inattentive when they were injured. Under Workman's Compensation, employers pay into an insurance system that provides medical care and a certain percentage, usually up to two thirds of the worker's wages, as long as he can't work.

A Larger Safety Net

If you don't qualify for this program, there are two other alternatives. If you develop health problems, regardless of their cause, but are now unable to work, you can apply for Social Security Disability Insurance (SSDI). Funded and managed by the Social Services Act, it provides a monthly cash allowance, as well as medical and hospital coverage through Medicare if you are totally disabled. In order to qualify for SSDI, you need to have been employed five out of the last ten years, contributing to the plan through deductions from your wages.

If you don't meet the five-year work requirement, then you can apply for Supplemental Security Income (SSI). You still need to establish that your health problems make it impossible to work, but you don't need to demonstrate that your work caused your illness or that you meet the five-year work standard. Both these programs also provide Medicare and Medicaid health benefits, depending on your circumstances.

Neither SSDI or SSI can be considered financial windfalls. The average SSDI monthly check varies from state to state and averages $600–700. SSI is significantly less, with an average of $300–400.

Going to Court

I never thought of the play *Macbeth* as a health risk until I met Carole Young. An actress who had trained at the Royal Academy of Dramatic Art in London, she came to me with sudden, severe asthma. Her problems began when she was cast as one of the three witches in a production of *Macbeth*. Apparently, the chemicals used in the boiling caldron as "double, double, toil and trouble" caused her to develop reactive airways dysfunction syndrome (RADS), a form of occupational airway disease. This distinct form of chronic airway obstruction typically begins with exposure to a very high concentration of an irritating chemical or gas. Breathing problems develop rapidly. With treatment, there is a gradual improvement, but lung function may not return to normal. Wheezing, cough, and shortness of breath continue, making it difficult to pursue a normal life. Although there can be no history of allergies, asthmatic attacks can become a long-term problem.

As an actress who, like most, was intermittently employed, Carole could not meet the requirements for SSDI because of the work history requirements. She was potentially eligible for Workman's Compensation. Believing, however, that the manufacturers of the chemicals used in the special effects of the caldron should take more responsibility for her continuing health problems that left her breathless and weak, she brought a lawsuit against the company that manufactured the chemicals. When she meets them in court, she will have to prove that the manufacturers marketed their product knowing the health risks involved and were negligent in protecting her safety.

Court action was also an option for Lydia Perez. In her early thirties, Lydia was living in a third-floor apartment in a walkup building in upper Manhattan. On a cold night in early March, the ancient boiler in her building cracked, causing a smoky fire. Lydia and the other tenants had complained for weeks about the smell of fuel oil and the piles of rags in the basement. Now the worst had happened. The building had burned and Lydia and her neighbors were not only homeless but had also suffered smoke inhalation. Two months later when Lydia came to see me, she was audibly wheezing. Once a healthy, active young woman, she was now a frequent visitor to the emergency room with severe asthmatic attacks. After several months, she realized she couldn't go back to work in the near future. She felt that the negligence of her landlord caused her health problems and sought compensation for the loss of her income, as well as the pain and suffering she had endured.

I am not advocating filing lawsuits whenever respiratory problems develop. But situations do arise where negligence has created health problems that radically change your life, and re-dress in the courts is clearly an option to explore.

Healthy Travel and Leisure

Angus Tucker was a man women loved and men admired. I would watch in awe as this self-made millionaire would skillfully handle his former wives and girlfriends as they paraded into his hospital room. Angus had been coming to see me for his COPD for five years, when I got a frantic call from a Florida hospital. Angus had been on a small plane, traveling to his home in the Keys, when he suddenly found he could not breathe. He was taken off the plane by stretcher, and was now on oxygen in a sunny Key West hospital.

I was concerned but not surprised. Air travel has a long list of drawbacks. Endless delays, long lines for security, frightening food, and seats designed for munchkins. For people without underlying pulmonary problems, stale cabin air causes headaches, sore throats, and itchy eyes. But for people with underlying respiratory problems, planes carry additional hazards. For Angus, the pressure in the small air cabin was low enough in oxygen to tax his already struggling respiratory system. In the future, I recommended that Angus use supplemental oxygen for plane travel.

Many health problems of air travel may start with the air quality in the cabin of the plane. It is a controversial and hotly debated issue. On one side is the airline industry, which stoutly maintains that cabin air is cleaner than the air found in the average home. They point to a Department of Transportation study that found levels of bacteria and fungi in the air of planes equal to or lower than that measured within the average private home. Airline industry spokespeople claim twenty to thirty complete air changes occur per hour. Since top-functioning

HEPA filters offer ten complete room air exchanges per hour, this is indeed an impressive statistic.

On the other side of the issue are the passengers, who know how they feel after a flight. They are joined by the flight attendants, whose union has repeatedly claimed that poor cabin air quality is causing health problems for its members.

At the core of the argument is the way air is circulated and filtered on a plane. In most modern jets, outside air is continuously drawn into the engines. This air is passed through a compressor and a portion of the compressed air is drawn off. It is then drawn into the air-conditioning system, where it is filtered and cooled. This air is mixed with equal parts of recycled air from the cabin and the mixture is reintroduced into the cabin. Some airlines and airplane manufacturers such as United and Boeing, point with pride to their use of HEPA air filters in their air-cleaning systems. Other, but certainly not all, airlines use these very efficient particulate filters.

How Fresh Is Fresh Enough?

The fifty/fifty mix is a figure that is under debate. Industry officials would like to change this balance to include a greater amount of the less expensive recirculated vs. the fresh compressed air. The reason for this is that it takes additional fuel, and thus additional money, to run the air-conditioning continuously at these high mixing levels. Passenger advocacy groups have been joined by the Association of Flight Attendants (AFA) to lobby for an increase of the more expensive, fresh, compressed air into the cabin mix, and reduce the percentage of recycled cabin air.

The acknowledged authority on air quality standards is the American Society of Heating, Refrigerating and Air-Conditioning Engineers (ASHRAE). This association established fresh air circulation standards for public buildings as fifteen cubic feet per person per minute (cfm). In planes, current ASHRAE standards recommend no less than ten cfm. Airline executives are lobbying hard to cut these already low standards in half to five cfm.

There is also concern about the carbon dioxide levels in the cabin air. ASHRAE standards for public buildings are 1,000 parts per million (ppm). These standards are defined for an environment where there are no harmful levels of contaminants in air and at least 80 percent of people do not feel discomfort. Even the airlines themselves admit that CO_2 levels in the planes can be routinely higher, at 1,500 ppm. Carbon dioxide pollution can cause headache and chest tightness.

Move It or Lose It

Cramped seats and enforced inactivity on a plane can also lead to blood clots in the veins of your legs. These clots can break off and flip into your lungs, where they cause pulmonary embolism. The seated position obstructs blood flow in the leg veins. This sluggish circulation is made worse by lack of leg muscle activity during a flight, which also keeps blood flowing through the body. If you have underlying heart disease, it is important that you get up and walk around every hour.

As a pulmonary physician, I am especially concerned about the low humidity in airplanes. Air moisture levels are usually between 15 and 20 percent and can drop to 6–10 percent during a long flight. This degree of air dryness is particularly troublesome for my patients with asthma because dry air cools the airway, causing cold-induced bronchospasm.

If you are sensitive to dogs and cats, call ahead to make sure no fellow passengers will be traveling with pets, as they can contribute to air quality problems. The allergens shed by the pets are circulated for the duration of the trip.

Do Drink the Water

Keep your body well-hydrated and drink eight oz. of cold bottled water every hour of the flight. Keep in mind that alcohol is dehydrating and carbonated beverages will make you feel bloated. On a short flight, do not eat the very salty pretzels, which can increase breathing discomfort. If you are on a longer flight, order a low-sodium meal. Airlines tend to use heavily processed foods that are high in salt and sulfites. Try to bring in your own healthy foods, such as fruit, yogurt, and low-sodium crackers.

Securing Additional Help

Even under ideal travel conditions, when there are underlying respiratory problems, you may feel increased shortness of breath on a plane. The higher altitudes mean reduced levels of oxygen in the cabin. Lower oxygen means that the lungs have to work harder to bring the same amount of oxygen to the rest of the body. Try using a short-acting bronchodilator if you experience chest tightness to provide relief during the flight. If your lung problems require oxygen supplementation during the day, you will require oxygen during the flight.

For safety and security reasons, airlines do not allow passengers to use their own oxygen. They will provide you with the necessary equipment. You will need a written request from your physicians at least forty-eight hours before your flight. The airlines will provide oxygen for each leg of the flight. The charge is usually in the $75–150 range, depending on the airline and the length of the flight.

A Healthier Flight

Sitting for hours on a plane that has been delayed for hours on a runway, you can feel like you have little control over the travel experience. Not completely true. There are six key ways that you can affect the health impact of your travel plans:

- Use your short-acting inhaler just before you board the plane.
- Travel early in the day when the planes are cleaner.
- Try to book a window seat in the front of the plane, where the air is reportedly fresher. (Window seats are closest to the air vents.)
- If the air starts to feel warm, ask the flight attendant to turn up the air-conditioning. The cooler temperatures are a sign of fresher air.
- Open the overhead air vents and keep them on for the duration of the trip.
- Carry all the medication you need in your briefcase or handbag and store them in the seat in front of you, not overhead.

A Healthy Home Away from Home

When you arrive at the hotel, ask for a nonsmoking, pet-free room. Try to avoid turning on blowers of the central heating and cooling system. The ducts can be blowing spores and pollutants into your room. If you find down pillows on the bed, ask housekeeping to replace them with foam bedding. If you are particularly sensitive to indoor pollution, think about carrying a small portable HEPA air-cleaning device. Place it on the nighttable on the side of the bed where you sleep.

Chapter 12

Effective Answers for Important Questions

The majority of patients in my practice share the same basic symptoms of asthma and COPD, but each one has individual questions and concerns. Since these pulmonary conditions are long-term problems, many of their concerns deal with lifestyle issues. Sometimes I can answer the questions easily, while other questions send me to the library or Internet for the best answers. I believe there is no such thing as a stupid question. Finding the answers has made me a better doctor, better able to help my patients manage their own respiratory health.

Smoking

Q: *My uncle smoked cigarettes every day of his long and healthy life until he died at the age of ninety. Are some people "immune" to the effects of tobacco smoke?*

A: Immune is a very strong word. We know that not everybody who smokes develops all of the complications that are associated with cigarettes. For example, only 15 to 20 percent of smokers develop chronic obstructive lung disease. Your uncle might have been one of the winners of the lucky gene pool that simply does not succumb to the toxic effects of tobacco. But those winners are few and far between. For every cigar-smoking George Burns who worked until he was ninety, there are ten Gracie Allens, who died of lung cancer when she was in her fifties.

Q: *I haven't smoked for ten years. Can I still get COPD?*

A: Unfortunately, yes. However, it is much less likely. It depends on how much damage there was before you gave up smoking, how long you smoked, and on the number of pack years that you have accumulated. It also depends on whether or not you get frequent respiratory infections, because those can accelerate the course of COPD.

Q: *I'm pregnant, and my husband smokes. Is this bad for the baby?*

A: Yes, in many ways. First of all, it can lead to the premature death of the father. In addition, studies have shown a relationship between secondhand smoke and low birth weight in babies. Babies that are smaller than anticipated at birth are at increased risk for lower IQ, hyperactivity, and congenital malformations. Cigarette smoking in the home before birth has also been linked to an increase in Sudden Infant Death Syndrome. As they grow older, children show lower lung function in a home with cigarette smoke. And children whose parents smoke are more likely to take up smoking, too.

Q: *I used to be a heavy smoker. Should I be getting a yearly CAT scan?*

A: No official agency or association has made that recommendation yet, but many pulmonologists are beginning to refer smokers over age fifty for an annual CAT scan of the chest. At the very least, I like to get a baseline CAT scan in my smoking patients over fifty to learn if there are any suspicious nodules on the lungs.

Q: *How can I get my teenage daughter to stop smoking?*

A: Teenagers can use nicotine replacement patches and gums to help wean them off cigarettes. Zyban may be valuable, since teenagers often have mood swings that seem to define adolescence. Without help, the anxiety of nicotine withdrawal is more than we can expect a teenager to manage. Remember that it is very hard for someone to quit in a home where an adult is a smoker. If cigarettes are not available in the home, then it is much less likely that she is going to have easy access, and much less likely that she will start smoking in the first place.

Q: *I've never smoked cigarettes, but my doctor now tells me that I have obstructive lung disease. How can this be?*

A: There are a number of situations that can lead to obstructive lung disease, even if you're not personally a smoker. For example, if you live or work with someone who smokes, it has been established that you can develop COPD from this secondhand smoke. If you have alpha-1 antitrypsin deficiency, it's possible to get COPD, even without cigarette smoking. In this hereditary disease, the patient lacks the protective factor in the blood, alpha-1 antitrypsin, that prevents white blood cells in your lung from digesting and destroying lung tissue every time an inflammation occurs. This leads to premature emphysema in persons less than fifty years of age. Additionally, we do know that many asthmatics go on to lose lung function as their asthma persists.

Q: *Since nicotine has such a bad effect on the heart, is it safe to use the patch or the gum?*

A: It's true that nicotine, one of the major toxicants in cigarette smoke, affects the heart. It speeds up heart rate and causes damage to the lining of the arteries. On the other hand, the amount of nicotine that you get from the nicotine replacement is designed to get progressively smaller and smaller, and eventually it is withdrawn altogether. Even though there may still be some continued risk from using a nicotine patch while you're coming off cigarettes, overall you're much better off trying to stop, even with the nicotine patch.

Q: *If I don't inhale, will smoking be less dangerous?*

A: This is a dangerous fallacy. The smoke from cigarettes still affects the upper airways. The mouth, throat, and nose can all be sites of cancers. Even though you don't make a conscious effort not to inhale it, some of the smoke still gets into the lungs. The smoke still billows around your face as you blow it out, and when you breathe in again, you're still breathing all those toxicants. It's at least as bad as secondhand smoke and probably a lot worse.

Q: *I've smoked for twenty years. Is it too late for me to quit?*

A: It's never too late to quit smoking. If you quit smoking and you're healthy, there's a good chance that you reduce your risk for many of the problems that cigarette smoking causes. If you already have some signs of cigarette-related disease, the progression of that disease may be slowed or even stopped by quitting smoking.

COPD

Q: *Does COPD increase my risk of developing lung cancer?*

A: These are two related problems that are linked to chronic airway irritation from cigarette smoke. As a result, many patients who are diagnosed with lung cancer also have chronic obstructive pulmonary disease. These days we're also discovering that people with COPD, who we didn't suspect of having lung cancer, do have malignant tumors. We're looking much more closely at these people, using CAT scans more frequently to identify specific areas of airway damage from COPD. Additionally, some patients with emphysema are going for chest surgery (frequently lung reduction surgery), and as a result of that surgery, we're finding unexpected small cancers in the lung. You need to remember that COPD, especially in the form of chronic bronchitis, is essentially a chronic irritation of the airways—and chronic irritation of anything frequently leads to cancer.

Q: *Are women more susceptible to COPD?*

A: Unfortunately, it may be true. Studies have shown that women smokers have lower lung function rates than men who have smoked the same number of pack years. Research has also demonstrated that women have a greater degree of airway hyperactivity. Doctors have suggested that a woman's naturally smaller lungs and airways increase their susceptibility to the damaging effects of cigarette smoking.

Q: *My mother died of COPD. Does that mean that I will get it, too?*

A: Not necessarily. Although you probably have a higher than average risk for COPD, the most important risk factor for COPD is not the genetic and health legacy of your parents, but your own smoking and lifestyle habits. Even if you have inherited an alpha-1 antitrypsin deficiency, if you stay away from cigarettes, you will probably avoid developing serious lung problems. In addition, following pulmonary protective strategies, such as an environmentally healthy home, a diet high in antioxidants, and quick treatment of colds and flus, will keep you and your lungs in the best possible shape.

Q: *Why does every cold I get turn into a heavy, lingering cough?*

A: Respiratory infections irritate the airways, damage the surface covering of the airways, and, as a result, the airways become even more hypersensitive than they normally are. This is why it is so important to aggressively treat colds before they can trigger an acute exacerbation of asthma or COPD.

Q: *My doctor told me my lung function is 50 percent, but I still feel pretty good. Did he do the test wrong?*

A: Not necessarily. The lung is a tremendously efficient organ, and unless you are a competitive athlete, 50 percent of lung function is usually enough to carry out many daily activities. Of course, it makes a difference whether you lost that other

50 percent over a short or a long period of time. If you lose the 50 percent quickly, you will certainly feel a decline in your health and fitness.

Q: *Should I see an allergist or a chest specialist for my breathing problems?*

A: It depends on the nature of your symptoms. Usually, patients with chronic bronchitis or emphysema see pulmonary specialists. Patients with upper respiratory allergies or those with mild asthma tend to be equally divided between ear-nose-and-throat doctors, pulmonary doctors who specialize in asthma, and allergists. Upper respiratory allergies, such as allergic rhinitis (hay fever), tend to respond to desensitization treatment, and that's something generally only an allergist provides. If you have severe asthma, it is probably wisest to consult with a pulmonologist.

Q: *When should I get a second opinion?*

A: Whenever you're not satisfied or comfortable with your first opinion. There's no shame or disgrace in getting a consultation with another physician. The real shame is missing a correct diagnosis. If you have a serious medical illness and you're not comfortable with the diagnosis or treatment that your doctor has given you, or you feel that there may be something else that needs to be said, then, by all means, seek a second opinion.

Lifestyle

Q: *Why do I start to wheeze in restaurants?*

A: You may have what we call "Restaurant Asthma," which is caused by a reaction to sulfites that are often added to commercial food preparations. Sulfites are effective antibacterial preservatives that extend the shelf life of foods and prevent spoilage and discoloration. Sulfites are routinely added to raw shrimp, wine, dried fruits, processed potatoes, fruit toppings, and vinegar, especially in foods prepared for restaurants.

Some asthmatics are particularly sensitive to these ingredients and can develop symptoms that range from simple asthma to a full-blown anaphylactic reaction when they're exposed to it. Doctors speculate that as sulfites are digested they release sulfur dioxide (SO_2 is one of the known major air pollutants in our environment). Other experts feel that there may be a true allergy to sulfites, involving IgE antibody formation. We also suspect that some asthmatics don't seem to have enzymes that break down sulfites efficiently.

Q: *Are alcoholic beverages good or bad for asthma/COPD?*

A: Wines that contain sulfites can precipitate bronchospasm in people with sensitive airways. If you feel shortness of breath after a few sips of wine, be sure you buy and drink sulfite-free wines, available from both California and New York State vineyards. Small amounts of alcohol in a cup of hot tea will not cause a problem, but excessive, regular alcohol consumption can be an irritant to your upper airways.

Questions have also been raised about the fermentation products in wine and beer. If you develop symptoms after a few sips, clearly these beverages are not for you. If a glass of wine or beer does not cause shortness of breath or upper airway congestion, these items should not be a problem for your respiratory system. But remember, excess alcohol consumption is as much of a killer as tobacco smoke.

Q: *Can wool blankets provoke asthma symptoms?*

A: Wool is an organic compound and a potential allergen. Wool blankets can indeed provoke allergies and asthma in sensitive people. So can wool carpeting, which will release irritating fibers in the air every time you walk on them. In addition, wool is particularly favored by dust mites, whose allergens are responsible for far too many episodes of nighttime breathing problems.

Q: *Can a menthol rub help ease my breathing?*

A: Mentholated rubs can loosen mucous secretions in the upper airways, which relieves nasal congestion. However, mentholated rubs often contain salicylates, which can be a problem if you have aspirin sensitivity.

About 10 percent of asthmatics have an aspirin intolerance. Aspirin relieves pain by blocking prostaglandin production, an inflammatory mediator (that is part of the arachidonic acid cascade). When inflammation occurs, the membrane that surrounds the cells of the body affected by the inflammation is damaged and releases arachinic acid. This molecule is then metabolized to a number of inflammatory mediators, such as the prostaglandins and leukotrienes, which cause painful swelling and redness. In some asthmatics, inhibition of prostaglandins produces a surge in leukotrienes, which are even more potent mediators for hypersensitive airways. Leukotrienes cause everything that you don't want to happen to airways, including bronchospasm, mucus production, and increase in white blood cells.

Q: *Will I gain weight if I eat all of the foods you recommend on the DASH diet?*

A: If you're a woman, you can reduce daily intake to six servings of grains, one serving of protein, and three servings of fruits. Make sure that the protein and dairy products you use are low-fat or fat-free. Carefully weigh protein servings and keep a close eye on fat portions. Keep in mind that the DASH diet is low in fat and sugar, which are the most highly concentrated sources of calories. You will be eating more food, but it will contain a lot less calories than the average American diet.

Q: *Should I move to a place like Arizona for my lungs?*

A: In a warm, dry place like Arizona, the chances of wintertime respiratory infections are significantly lower. In a cold climate, the air itself may cause bronchospasm. Also, the cold, wet weather keeps people indoors, where there's a lot more transmission of infection. Some experts argue that by moving to a warm, dry climate, you move away from industrial centers of the country to a place where there may be less air pollution. On the downside, many of these warmer climates have new types of vegetation, new fauna, and new flora. If you have allergies as a basis of your chronic lung disease, then such a move may actually make your breathing problems worse. My advice to anyone who is contemplating such a move is to "let the buyer beware." Try out the climate before you make a commitment. Visit during different seasons to gauge how the climate affects you at different times of the year. Keep in mind that moving to another climate also means leaving most of your friends and family support system.

Q: *I try to escape the winter cold by going to Florida, but each time I go, I get more asthmatic attacks. Is this just a coincidence?*

A: It may be a coincidence, but I hear this so frequently from my patients that I have to think that Florida may not be the ideal vacation spot if you have chronic lung disease. Many patients with chronic lung disease are sensitive to the types of flora and fauna that are found in hot, humid climates, and as a result, their breathing gets much worse.

Q: *Should I use a humidifier?*

A: Separating my patients from their humidifiers is almost as difficult as separating them from their pets. It is true that dry, cold air dries out mucous membranes and makes it harder to get rid of phlegm in the airways, but room humidifiers are not the answer.

For optimum health, the humidity in a home or apartment should be kept between 40 and 50 percent. Higher humidity levels encourage unhealthy levels of bacteria, allergens, and pollen in the home environment. A number of my patients like to run their bedroom humidifier all night with their windows and door shut. By morning, they could practically grow orchids in the room. High levels of humidity encourage the growth of mold and dust mites, while pollutants dissolve in the moisture laden air, waiting to be inhaled.

There are four types of humidifiers, and I have problems with three of them. The *ultrasonic* or *cool mist* humidifier uses sound energy to produce minute droplets of water from the humidifier reservoir water tank. These droplets are then blown in a stream out of the machine. Problems arise when bacteria, mold, and algae, which accumulate in the tank of water, are aerosolized into your home. It is necessary to scrub out the tank daily to avoid contamination, and then you stand the risk of aerosolizing traces of the cleaning fluids. Old-fashioned *steam* humidifiers have similar problems aerosolizing contaminants. In addition, they can tip over and inflict a painful burn. *Evaporative pad* humidifiers operate by blowing air across a wet mesh pad to pick up moisture. These pads are an open invitation for bacteria and fungus to make a home. The *warm mist* humidifiers boil water to create moisture, which is cooled before the mist is introduced into the room. They also contain a humidity-sensing control device that shuts the machine off when the room humidity rises to a preset level. If you feel you must have a humidifier, this is the model I would choose.

I believe that it is safer and more effective to humidify yourself. If your nose and chest feel congested, take a long hot shower. Humidify your body with plenty of hot and cold fluids, such as tea, chicken soup, and water.

Q: *Do ionizers clean the air?*
A: Ionizers generate ions that charge airborne pollutant parti-

cles and pull them out of the atmosphere in your home. Nevertheless, some particles settle on walls or furniture and can be released when people start moving around a room. Additionally, the ionizer's filter tends to quickly become clogged with debris and no longer cleans the air. When they are cleaned, particles can be released back into the air. Older models tend to give off ozone, which can irritate even healthy normal airways. In general, we prefer using HEPA filter air purifiers, which remove the particles from the air simply by trapping them in their filters.

Q: *What is the best type of face mask used to avoid pollution?*

A: Most face masks are not very effective. If they don't fit tightly, pollutants are still inhaled into your airways. When they have a suitably tight fit, most of my patients find they make breathing very difficult. If there is air pollution or a pollen alert, my best advice is to stay indoors with the windows closed and the air conditioner and HEPA air purifiers running.

Q: *I have chronic bronchitis, and my neighbor says I shouldn't use hair spray. Is she right?*

A: Yes. It's been shown that hair sprays can be irritating to the airway, and people with asthma/COPD can develop spasms of their airways as a result of breathing in the aerosolized chemicals that those products contain. In addition, many of the toiletries and household-cleaning aerosols that we use are either scented or contain irritating chemicals. Pump sprays may be kinder to the environment, but are still a problem for sensitive airways. Always look for products that are applied directly.

Q: *The house I want to buy has an asbestos wrapping around the pipes and furnace. Should I still make an offer?*

A: Almost every house built before 1976 can have asbestos in one form or another, so it's hard to make a unilateral statement. You should have the house inspected by somebody who knows what they're looking for. As a rule of thumb, if the insulation that is surrounding your heating system or plumbing is in good condition and there is no sign of asbestos dust, it's probably better not to have it removed. Decontamination may cause more problems than leaving it alone. If the insulation is cracked and flaky, then you may need to reconsider your options. And never try to remove the asbestos yourself. This is definitely not a Home Depot weekend project. You can seriously contaminate your home and damage your lungs.

Q: *Does steam cleaning do a better job of cleaning wall-to-wall carpets?*

A: I think steam cleaning and carpets are words that shouldn't be in the asthmatic/COPD vocabulary. Wall-to-wall carpets act as a reservoir for living and dead irritants, and steam cleaning will dislodge those irritants into the air. In addition, steam cleaning can leave the carpet slightly damp, which can lead to the growth of molds. If you have carpeting that needs steam cleaning, you already are causing problems for yourself, and steam cleaning is definitely not the solution.

Allergy and Asthma

Q: *I have had scoliosis since I was a teenager. Now my doctor tells me that this old problem is complicating my asthma. How did this happen?*

A: Scoliosis causes a lung problem that is a separate issue from asthma, but can complicate it. Scoliosis causes what we call restriction, which means an inability of the lungs to take a deep breath. As scoliosis progresses, restriction increases. This means that, in addition to having difficulty moving air through the airways from asthma, there's difficulty moving the chest in general. The severity of the scoliosis is determined by the shape of the back—in other words, how much the spine curves as it twists. For the majority of people who have scoliosis (and most of these turn out to be women), the problem is minimal and has little effect on breathing. For the 5 to 10 percent for whom scoliosis is severe, this can produce serious, even life-threatening, problems.

Q: *Why can't my doctor find the cause of my asthma?*
A: It turns out that most asthmatics are sensitive to a wide variety of irritants. It may not be possible to completely eliminate all allergens and triggers in your environment, but diligence should reduce the severity and frequency of symptoms.

Q: *I used to have asthma as a child. How can I prevent it in my son?*
A: Make sure your home is a smoke-free environment. Not only is secondhand smoke a dangerous irritant, but most serious smokers grew up with parents who smoked. Secondly, at the risk of sounding cruel, I advise a pet-free environment. Pets are highly allergenic and increase your son's chances of developing antibodies that provoke asthmatic airways. Paradoxically, a study published in the fall of 2002 in the *New England Journal of Medicine* suggests that children exposed to pets in the first year of life actually had reduced

risks of developing allergies. However, it is important to re-member that there are a number of studies that indicate pets introduced after the age of one are still linked to allergies in families where there is a history of sensitivities.

In your home, follow principles of pulmonary protective housekeeping: Use HEPA filters in room purifiers, air con-ditioners, and vacuum cleaners, and put dust mite protective coverings on all beds and upholstered furniture. Finally, make sure your son gets all his vaccines on schedule and treat sniffles and colds aggressively to prevent permanent airway damage.

Q: *Are some breeds of dogs less allergenic than others?*

A: Not really. In theory, the hairless or short hair dogs, like Jack Russell terriers or dachshunds, are less allergenic. But if you're sensitive to dogs, it's likely that even these dogs are going to cause allergic reactions, because it is not just the dander in the pet hair that causes bronchoconstriction. Dog urine and saliva are also high in allergens that provoke respi-ratory problems.

Q: *Does the hairless cat cause less of a problem with allergies?*

A: Not all of the allergens are carried in the hair. Cat saliva and urine are also sources of allergens, so you can be very aller-gic to even a hairless cat.

Q: *Should I avoid down bedding?*

A: In a word, yes. The Latin species name for dust mites trans-lates to "feather-loving" . . . mites love eating feathers. Feath-ers can also break down and the little particles can become aerosolized. When inhaled, these sharp particles can irritate your lungs. Also keep in mind that feathers are outright allergens, stimulating overproduction of IgE antibodies.

Remember that there is also a lot of down in good quality chairs and couches. Many hotels have down pillows, and some of my patients report that they suffer increased respiratory problems on holiday and business trips. When you check into a hotel, always ask if they use down pillows. Request foam bedding for a trouble-free stay.

Alternative Health

Q: *I don't like fish. Can I take omega-3 fish oil supplements?*

A: Studies have shown that two or more weekly servings of fish are linked to a reduction in risk of COPD or asthma. When researchers tried using just fish oil supplements, there was no change in respiratory health. If you don't like fish, there are other ways that you can control the pulmonary problems, but fish supplements will not give you the benefits you're looking for.

Q: *Should I add more soy to my food?*

A: Research has shown significant health benefits from soy protein. Soy can lower cholesterol levels, which reduces the risk of heart disease. In addition, soy is felt to lower the risk of certain types of breast cancer. Although soy has not been shown to affect pulmonary health, its wide-ranging benefits can strengthen overall well-being.

Q: *Can Chinese herbs help my breathing?*

A: Chinese herbal preparations for asthma usually contain Ma-Huang, a bush that contains large amounts of ephedrine.

The problem with herbal combinations is that you don't know their potency or whether they have been modified. Sometimes the Chinese herbs have been adulterated with theophylline or steroids to make them more effective so they could be too strong, making you nauseous or causing a rapid heartbeat that could be fatal. Alternatively, they could be too weak and not relieve your bronchospasm.

Q: *What vitamins should I be taking?*

A: I recommend a multivitamin for everyone. If you are dealing with a chronic disease such as asthma/COPD, two multivitamins per day will provide extra coverage. At this point, there is no recommendation for single, additional supplements, because studies have shown that they don't work and in some cases can increase your risk for lung cancer.

Q: *I get symptoms of hypoglycemia from fruit. Why can't I get my vitamins from supplements?*

A: Unless you have uncontrolled diabetes, fresh fruit, especially if it's taken as part of the meal, should not cause wild fluctuations in your blood sugar levels. Supplements don't provide the protection seen in diets rich in fruits and vegetables. If you get hungry between meals, try eating a vegetable salad, rather than fruit, as a snack.

Q: *Can acupuncture help asthma?*

A: There are some studies that show that acupuncture by a trained practitioner can produce relief equivalent to that of a low dose of a short-acting bronchodilator. If you want to use acupuncture along with your medication, it can provide some symptomatic relief. The danger occurs when people try to use acupuncture instead of their medication because acupuncture alone doesn't deal with inflammation, which is the underlying cause of asthma and the long-term changes in lung structure. If you want to use acupuncture, add it to your existing treatment plan. Don't use it instead of medication.

Q: *Will a cup of hot tea, honey, and lemon help my breathing?*

A: Tea contains small amounts of theophylline, which relaxes bronchospasm. Hot vapors from the tea can moisturize the phlegm that may be in your upper airway, so you will be able to cough it up or blow your nose so that you can clear your sinuses a bit. The honey coats the mucous membranes, protecting them from irritation. But this soothing hot beverage should be used in addition to, not instead of, your usual medication.

Medications

Q: *Will inhaled steroids give me "chipmunk cheeks"?*

A: Well, there is some controversy on this point. Over the years, we have been moving to higher and higher doses of more potent inhaled steroids, and there is increasing evidence that some of these steroids when inhaled may be absorbed into the body, leading to the same swelling of the face that is one of the consequences of using oral steroids. Fortunately, these consequences are usually much less severe than they are with oral steroids.

Q: *Will inhaled steroids give me osteoporosis?*

A: That is one of the things that is now being studied. We're using much higher doses, and there are signs that these doses are being absorbed, so there may be side effects along those lines. It's now prudent for women past menopause to track bone density when they use inhaled steroids.

Q: *Won't inhaled steroids give me facial hair and acne?*

A: Inhaled steroids have the potential for all the side effects seen in either oral or injected steroids, but by and large, their side effects are less.

Q: *I took a flu shot, but I still got the flu. What happened?*

A: The flu vaccination is not an infallible form of protection. The flu vaccine is prepared before the influenza epidemic or season begins, so it's only a guess as to which particular virus is going to be the flu virus of the year. In addition, many people complain that they have developed the flu, when in fact they are suffering from a bad upper respiratory infection with a run-of-the-mill cold virus. Since we don't usually test for the exact type of virus that you have, it's usually a guessing game as to whether or not the flu vaccine has worked in you or not.

Q: *Can I still get pneumonia after I get the pneumonia shot?*

A: Yes, you can. The pneumonia vaccine, which is good for five to ten years, protects you against more than twenty strains of bacteria that cause strep pneumonia, the most common form of bacterial pneumonia. However, there are other forms of bacterial or viral pneumonia which can occur.

Pneumonia vaccines are used primarily for people who are more susceptible, either because of their age or because of their immune status. You should realize the average American has a 1 in 100 chance of developing pneumonia each year, and this vaccine considerably improves your odds of staying healthy.

Q: *How do I know when to replace my inhaler?*

A: Generally, the standard canister contains about 200 puffs. If you use it four times a day, with two puffs for each treatment, that's eight puffs a day. At this rate, an inhaler should last about three weeks. If you lose track of time, put the canister in a bowl of water. If only half of the canister is still above the waterline, it is almost empty and you need to refill your prescription.

Q: *Should I use a powder or a liquid inhaler?*

A: We are now moving more toward powder inhalers for several reasons: Powders are more environmentally friendly, since they don't contain chlorofluorocarbons that deplete the ozone layer. With powders, you can accurately measure how much medication you are taking because you either have to load the powder delivery system with a single dose each time you use it, or there's an indicator on the container that tells you how many more doses are left. And finally, powder delivery systems are designed to require less coordination of the patient to use them. You don't have to coordinate the squeezing of the canister with the inhalation of the powder, so you're more likely to inhale all the required medication.

Q: *Should I use a nebulizer?*

A: Generally, we recommend nebulizers for our sicker patients, as they can deliver more medication, and they can deliver it in a fashion that doesn't require as much coordination from the patient. With a nebulizer, you just breathe naturally, rather than having to coordinate your inhalation with an inhaler. Consequently, we're more confident that the medicine is being delivered. If your doctor suggests one, you should know there are now some battery-powered nebulizers that are small enough to put in your pocket and take with you.

Q: *Why has my medication stopped working?*

A: The easiest reason to think of is that there's no more medication in your inhaler. (Some inhalers now come with an indicator of how much medication is left in your inhaler.) Another possibility is that you've gotten sicker and obstruction has increased. So you now have to either use more of it to get the same effect, or you have to add new drugs to your treatment plan. Another reason that people become less responsive to a medication is because they develop tachyphylaxis, a ten-dollar word that indicates resistance has developed to a medication. This may be a sign that we need to change medication or add new ones to the treatment plan.

Sodium Values
of Common Foods

Food	Milligrams of Sodium
½ cup canned peas	308
½ cup canned corn	170
½ cup canned mushrooms	536
½ cup fresh mushrooms	6
1 cup cooked kidney beans	2
½ cup canned baked beans	485
1 cup tomato juice	700
1 dill pickle	1900
1 fresh cucumber	14
1 slice of white bread	140
10 potato chips	70
1 cup corn flakes	325
3 pancakes	600
1 cup canned chicken noodle soup	1107
1 cup won ton soup	2027
1 cup tomato juice	365
1 tablespoon salted butter	150
1 tablespoon unsalted butter	7
½ cup ice cream	75
1 oz. cheddar cheese	198
1 cup whole milk	120

Food	Milligrams of Sodium
1 cup yogurt	117
1 cup instant breakfast	242
1 oz. of ham	312
1 cup cooked chili	1355
3 oz. canned tuna fish	535
1 frankfurter	776
1 oz. of bologna	370
Burger King Whopper with cheese	1164
KFC fried chicken breast	654
McDonald's Egg McMuffin	885
Taco Bell Burrito	922
⅔ cup Rice a Roni	820
1 cup macaroni and cheese	1085
1 bouillon cube	960
2 tablespoons of soy sauce	2665
1 tablespoon bottled Italian dressing	315

Resource Section

I have found that these organizations can be wonderful sources of informations on a wide range of issues important to people concerned about pulmonary problems. You can download up-to-the-minute information on their Web sites or call them to ask questions or to send specific information.

National Asthma Education and Prevention Program
NHLBI Information Center
301-592-8573
www.nhlbi.nih

American Lung Association of the City of New York
212-889-3370
www.alany.org

American Academy of Allergy, Asthma, and Immunology
800-822-2762
www.aaaai.org

Asthma and Allergy Foundation of America
800-727-8462
www.aafa.org

American College of Allergy, Asthma, and Immunology
800-842-7777
www.allergy.mcg.edu

Allergy and Asthma Network/Mothers of Asthmatics, Inc.
800-878-4403
www.podi.com/health/aanma

National Jewish Medical Research Center (Lung Line)
800-222-5864
www.njc.org

Health House Project
651-227-8014
www.healthhouse.org

Indoor Air Quality Information Clearinghouse
800-438-4318
www.epa.gov.iaq

National Air Duct Cleaners Association
202-737-2926
www.nada.com

American College of Chest Physicians
847-498-1400
www.chestnet.org

American Association of Respiratory Care
972-243-2273
www.aarc.org

Environmental Protection Agency
www.epa.gov

National Institute of Occupational Safety and Health
www.cdc.gov/niosh

Occupational Safety and Health Agency
www.OSHA.gov

American Thoracic Society
www.thoracic.org

Suppliers of Pulmonary Protective Products

AFM Enterprises Inc.
800-239-0321
www.afmsafecoat.com
Provides nonirritating paints and wood finishes

Achoo Allergy and Air Products
404-327-3100
www.achooallergy.com
Large catalog: air purifiers, bedding, cleaning products, vacuum
cleaners, window filters, dehumidifiers, masks, asthma management tools

Allergy Relief Shop, Inc.
800-626-2810
www.Allergyreliefshop.com
Source of nonirritating cleaning products, paints, and solvents

Allergy Store
954-472-0128
www.allergystore.com
Wide stock includes air filters, trickle ventilation, dust mite covers, and HEPA vacuum cleaners

Easy Breathe Ltd.
800-735-4772
www.easybreathe.com
Stock includes HEPA air cleaners, antimite bed coverings, and high-performance furnace filters

State Allergy
813-872-7844
www.stateallergy.com
Low-allergy cleaning supplies, vacuum cleaners

National Allergy Supply, Inc.
800-522-1448
www.nationalallergy.com
Items include a wide selection of antimite bedding, HEPA filters, and vacuum cleaners

Allersearch Labs
800-686-6483
Nonirritating cleaning products

Heart of Vermont
800-639-4123
www.heartofvermont.com
Bedding products for chemically sensitive and environmentally
aware

Mission: Allergy
877-662-5537
Informative color catalog with fabric sample of antimite bedding, as well as marks, vacuum cleaners, dehumidifiers, 3M air-
conditioning filters

The Filter Market
877-943-4587
www.filtermarket.com
Huge selection of high-quality furnace filters

ProLab
800-427-0550
www.prolabinc.com
Mold detection test kits

Manufacturers

If you have questions about a specific product or are looking for retail sources, you can contact the manufacturers directly.

Panasonic
800-211-PANA
HEPA air purifiers
www.panasonic.com

GlaxoSmithKline
888-825-5249
www.ibreathe.com
Advair, Serevent, Zyban, Flovent

Miele, Inc.
800-843-7231
www.miele.com
HEPA vacuum cleaners

Austin Air Systems, Ltd.
716-856-3700
Air purifiers

3M
www.3M.com/filtrete
Manufactures high-performance furnace filters and air-conditioning filters

Swiffer
Markets electrostatic dust cloths that pick up and remove allergens and dust
800-214-8734
www.swiffer.com

Whirlpool
Makes Whispure air purifiers with HEPA filters
866-878-4372 or 800-253-1301
www.whispure.com

Eureka
Affordable HEPA vacuum cleaners
www.eureka.com

Honeywell
800-332-1110
Affordable effective HEPA air filters
www.kaz.com

Smoking Cessation Support

These organizations and Web sites offer a wide range of materials to help you quit smoking.

American Cancer Society
800-227-2345
www.cancer.org

American Lung Association
800-586-4872
www.lungusa.org

American Heart Association
212-373-6300
www.amhrt.org

www.quitnet
Offers interactive system to record your programs, outlines for quitting, and tips like best ways to avoid weight gain when you quit

www.kickbutt.org
Offers valuable quitting strategies

www.drquit.com
Provides articles on how to quit, as well as chat rooms for support

Nicotine Anonymous
877-879-6422
www.nicotine-anonymous.org

Smokenders
1-800-828-4357
www.smokenders.com
Thirty-year-old program has helped more than 1 million people to quit

Nicorette.com
A Web site dedicated to information for using Nicorette to
stop smoking

Smoke Free
www.smokefree.org

www.habitrol.org
Provides online support groups and toll free talks with professional counselors

Publications

Asthma Magazine
1-800-654-2452

Allergy and Asthma Health
Official magazine of Allergy & Asthma Network/Mothers of
Asthmatics
www.aanma.org

Respiratory News and Previews
Excellent newsletter published by Asthma/Emphysema Self-
Help Group
212-777-0486

Glossary

adrenaline hormone isolated from the adrenal gland. Trademark for epinephrine, it is used in the treatment of asthma and anaphylaxis.

aerosol a fine spray of liquid particles that can hang in the air.

agonist a drug that attaches to a body cell receptor and causes the same action as the body's own natural agent.

airway hyperreactivity a key feature of asthma characterized by an exaggerated constriction of the airways to irritants.

alpha-1 antitrypsin the body's agent that prevents the enzyme elastase from overdigesting elastin in lung tissue.

alveoli the microscopic air sacs that are responsible for the transfer of oxygen and carbon dioxide into and out of the lungs. These are the structures that are damaged in emphysema.

anaphylaxis a severe, life-threatening allergic reaction.

antagonists drugs that attach to cell receptors but do not cause the response that is normally associated with the body's natural agent. Beta blockers are antagonists of Albuterol and epinephrine.

antigens foreign substances that provoke an allergic response.

antiprotease antienzyme that blocks action of enzymes that can destroy healthy tissue.

arachidonic acid chemical produced in the body during allergic or inflammatory response, which in turn leads to leukotrienes and prostaglandins, all of which lead to further airway distress.

asthma a chronic inflammation of the airways causing episodes of wheezing, breathlessness, chest tightness, and coughing.

beta blockers drugs used for heart disease and high blood pressure.

bioflavinoids a group of biologically active compounds found in plants, especially citrus fruits.

bronchi large airways in the lung that become inflamed and swollen in an asthmatic attack.

bronchioles small airways that become inflamed and damaged in asthma and other forms of COPD.

bronchoconstrictor a substance that causes the smooth muscles of the airway to contract, causing the airways to narrow.

bronchodilator medications such as beta 2 agonists and anticholinergic agents that relax the airways.

bronchospasm constriction of the airways.

catacholamines a group of drugs and natural hormones, related to the adrenal hormones epinephrine (adrenalin) and norepinephrine sharing the same basic structure.

cilia tiny hairlike structures on the surface of the airway cells that sweep dirt and bacteria out of the lungs.

chronic bronchitis a form of COPD where the bronchi are inflamed and clogged with excess mucus.

CO_2 carbon dioxide, a gas that is one of the end products of the cellular metabolism. It is transported by the blood from the body to the lungs, where it is eliminated in exhaled air. Inadequate ventilation that occurs in severe COPD leads to the accumulation of CO_2 in the blood.

cystic fibrosis a hereditary disease where the lungs produce large amounts of sticky, thick mucus. Symptoms of coughing and frequent respiratory infections, as well as malnutrition, appear in childhood, but milder cases may not be diagnosed until early adulthood.

elastase a natural enzyme that is produced by white blood cells that digests elastin fibers in the body.

EPA Environmental Protection Agency. An agency of the Federal Government established in 1970 to do research, monitor, and enforce standards set to regulate the environment.

epidemiology that branch of medicine that studies the causes and controls of diseases in large populations.

exacerbation a worsening of symptoms that calls for prompt medical attention.

FEV1 Forced Expiratory Volume in one second. The amount of air that you can forcefully blow out of your lungs in one second after a deep inhalation. This measurement falls as your airways become more constricted.

free radicals unstable, damaged molecules that lose an electron and can cause inflammation and cell damage.

HDL High-Density Lipoproteins. Proteins in the blood that transport fats and cholesterol. A high HDL is usually associated with a favorable cardiovascular profile.

Hippocratic Oath the pledge that doctors take when they graduate medical school, which reflects the ethical basis of the profession.

HVAC system stands for Heating, Ventilating, and Air-Conditioning system. It is the equipment that controls the environmental temperature and amount of air that is circulated in a home or workplace.

IgE antibodies produced by the body which cause many allergic reactions, such as those associated with hay fever and asthma. Some people who tend to produce greater quantities of IgE tend to have a number of allergies.

immunoglobulins antibodies.

irritant asthma asthma that results from exposure to irritant particles, aerosols, or gases.

isocyanates chemicals used in paints and plastics that can be irritating to the respiratory system.

isokinetic exercise use of exercise machines to work muscles through a complete range of motion.

LDL Low-Density Lipoprotein. Proteins in the blood that transport fats and cholesterol. A high LDL is usually associated with an increased risk of heart disease.

leukotrienes inflammatory cellular chemicals that play an important role in asthmatic attack. Allergens and free radicals promote the release of leukotrienes; there are now medications that block their effects and may reduce incidence of asthma attacks, particularly in children.

low-tar cigarettes tar in cigarettes has been linked to both cancer and heart disease. Low-tar tobacco that has been processed to lower tar levels may sound like a step in the right direction, but the concept is very misleading. People often compensate by taking deeper puffs and smoking more cigarettes.

occupational asthma a form of asthma caused by a specific agent or process present in the workplace.

ozone O_3 is an unstable, reactive gas that is one of the criteria pollutants formed by the reaction of automobile exhaust, oxygen in the atmosphere, and sunlight. Irritating to both healthy and troubled airways.

mediators substances, such as histamine or leukotrienes, released during an allergic reaction which cause inflammation.

mucus a viscous, elastic substance that is secreted by and coats the airway lining protecting it from inhaled irritants and infectious agents. (Mucous is the adjective that describes properties of mucus.)

NIOSH National Institute for Occupational Safety and Health. Federal agency responsible for conducting research and making recommendations for the prevention of work-related disease and injury. NIOSH is part of the Centers for Disease Control and Prevention (CDC).

NO_2 nitrogen dioxide. An irritating air pollutant that is one of the EPA's criteria pollutants. It is generated primarily by motor vehicle exhaust and stationary power sources such as electric power plants.

nutriceuticals vitamin supplements used as medication either to prevent or relieve disease.

OSHA Occupational Safety and Health Administration. A division of the Department of Labor responsible for creating and enforcing workplace safety and health regulations.

particulate form of air pollutant consisting of particles suspended in the air. The EPA designates this pollution as PM (particulate matter) and classifies it by size (less than 10 microns, less than 2.5 microns). Particles of this size have been associated with cardiovascular and pulmonary damage and with increased chance of dying.

peak flow maximum speed at which air can be exhaled after taking in a deep breath. Measured with a peak flow meter, a portable instrument, it is useful for monitoring lung function at home or in the workplace.

polyunsaturated fats from vegetables and nuts that were thought at one point to lower cholesterol and lower risk of heart disease.

prostaglandins mediators formed, in general following inflammation, as a result of the metabolism of arachidonic acid. Aspirin and other nonsteroidal anti-inflammatory drugs block this process.

RADS Reactive Airways Dysfunction Syndrome. Term used to describe a chronic obstructive airway disease resulting from an exposure to high concentrations of an environmental irritant, frequently in the workplace.

receptors specialized molecules that bind agonists, mediators, and drugs with a high degree of specificity initiating cellular actions such as smooth muscle constriction or relaxation.

rhinitis inflammation of the mucous membranes of the nose.

scurvy a disease resulting from vitamin C deficiency, characterized by weakness, anemia, and bleeding of the gums.

sinusitis inflammation of the sinuses, the air-filled cavities that are found in the bones of the skull.

SO$_2$ sulfur dioxide. A criteria pollutant of the EPA, irritating to persons with chronic airway disease, particularly asthmatics.

Formed as the result of burning fuels with a high sulfur content.

SSDI Social Security Disability Insurance. Insurance covering medical expenses for disabled workers and providing partial wage replacement during a worker's period of disability. It requires that the disabled worker have paid into the federally administered fund for at least five of the last ten years.

SSI Supplemental Security Income. Insurance covering medical expenses for disabled individuals, unable to work, and providing partial wage replacement during a worker's period of disability. Administered by both the State and Federal Government and funded through general taxes, it does not have a specific work history requirement for eligibility.

tachyphylaxis when a formerly effective medication no longer relieves symptoms in spite of adequate dosing.

tar particulates in cigarette smoke linked to cancer and heart disease.

wheeze high-pitched sound, heard either with or without a stethoscope, that corresponds to vibrations of the airway due to limitation of flow in a constricted airway.

Workman's Compensation No-fault insurance covering medical expenses for work-related injuries and providing partial wage replacement during a worker's period of disability. The insurance is usually paid for by the employer and administered through the State, except in the case of Federal and other special employees.

Bibliography

Books

Barnes, Peter (ed.): *Asthma*. 2nd ed. Academic Press (San Diego), 1998.

Barnes, Peter: *Managing Chronic Obstructive Pulmonary Disease*. Science Press (London), 2000.

Cherniack, Neil (ed.): *Chronic Obstructive Pulmonary Disease*. W. B. Saunders (Philadelphia), 1991.

Chiras, Daniel D.: *Environmental Science*. 2nd ed. Benjamin/Cummings (Menlo Park), 1988.

Committee on Passive Smoking. Board on Environmental Studies & Toxicology: *Environmental Tobacco Smoke*. National Academy Press (D.C.), 1986.

Fishman, Alfred (ed.): *Pulmonary Rehabilitation*. Marcel Dekker, Inc. (New York), 1996.

Frownfelter, Donna, et al: *Principles and Practical Cardiopulmonary Physical Therapy* 3rd ed. Mosby (St. Louis), 1996.

Haas, Francois, et al: *Pulmonary Therapy and Rehabilitation*. Williams & Wilkins (Philadelphia), 1991.

Hodgkin, John, et al (eds.): *Pulmonary Rehabilitation*. 3rd ed. Lippincott (Philadelphia), 2000.

Jones, Norman: *Clinical Exercise Testing.* 4th ed. W. B. Saunders (Philadelphia), 1997.

McDermott, Henry J.: *Handbook of Ventilation for Contaminant Control.* Butterworth Publishers (Boston), 1985.

National Cancer Institute: *Changes in Cigarette-Related Disease Risks and the Implications for Prevention and Control.* NIH Monograph, 1999.

National Cancer Institute: *Health Effects of Exposure to Environmental Tobacco Smoke.* NIH Monograph, 1999.

Niederman, Michael, et al: *Respiratory Infections.* 2nd ed. Lippincott, Williams & Wilkins (Philadelphia), 2001.

Ries, Andrew L., et al: *Shortness of Breath.* 6th ed. C. V. Mosby (St. Louis), 2001.

CHAPTER 1

George, Ronald B., et al: *Chest Medicine.* 4th ed. Lippincott, Williams & Wilkins (Philadelphia), 2000.

Hirsch, Albert, et al (ed.): *Prevention of Respiratory Diseases.* Marcel Dekker, Inc. (New York), 1993.

How to Help Patients Stop Smoking: Guidelines for Diagnosis and Treatment of Nicotine Dependence. AMA Division of Health Science.

Murray, C. J., Lopez, A.: *Alternative Projections of Mortality and Disability by Cause 1990–2020.* Global Burden of Disease Study. *The Lancet,* 1997; 349: 1436–42.

CHAPTER 2

Cassburi, Richard: *Principles & Practice of Pulmonary Rehabilitation.* W. B. Saunders (Philadelphia), 1993.

DesJardins, Terry: *Cardiopulmonary Anatomy and Physiology.* 4th ed. Delmar Publisher, 2002.

Fishman, Alfred, et al (ed.): *Pulmonary Diseases and Disorders.* McGraw Hill Book Co. (New York), 1998.

Weiss, Earle, et al: *Bronchial Asthma.* 3rd ed. Little, Brown (Boston), 1993.

CHAPTER 3

Advances in Asthma Management. Johns Hopkins University School of Medicine. Vol. 2, No. 1 (Jan.), 2002.

Asthma and Allergic Rhinitis: Connecting Common Pathways and Treatments. Internal Medicine World Report. Vol. 16, No. 11 (Oct.), 2001.

Briggs, Dick D., et al, The National COPD Awareness Panel: *Early Detection and Management of COPD. The Journal of Respiratory Diseases.* 21 (Sept., Vol. 21, No. 9A), 2000.

BTS Guidelines for the Management of Chronic Obstructive Pulmonary Disease. Thorax. 1997; 52 Suppl. 5: S1–S28.

Busse, William, Kumor, Aarna: *Recognizing and Controlling Exercise-Induced Asthma. The Journal of Respiratory Diseases.* 1995; 16: 1087–96.

Closing the Gender Gap: Women and COPD. American Thoracic Society Symposium Excerpts, 2001.

Cochrane, G. Mac, et al: *Asthma—Current Perspectives.* Mosby Nolte (London), 1996.

COPD, the Next New Killer Disease. Internal Medicine World Report. 2001.

Coultas, David: *The Health Impact of Undiagnosed Airflow Obstruction in a National Study of United States Adults. Am J Respir Crit Care Med.* 2001; 164: 372–77.

Expert Panel 2: Guidelines for the Diagnosis and Management of Asthma. NIH Publication. No. 97–4051, April 1997.

Facts About Home Control of Asthma and Allergies. ALA Pamphlet, 12/97.

Fischer, Andrew, et al: *Identifying and Treating Aspirin-Induced Asthma. J Resp Dis.* 1995; 16: 304–18.

Global Initiative for Asthma—Global Strategy for Asthma Management and Prevention. NHLBI/WHO Report, Revised 2002.

Gonzales, Ralph, et al: *Uncomplicated Acute Bronchitis. Ann Intern Med.* 2000; 133: 981–91.

Ground Zero: Assessing the Respiratory Impact. Pulmonary reviews. Jan. 2002. Vol. 7, No. 1, pp. 1–2.

Guidelines Spotlight Neglected COPD. Internal Medicine News. 2001; May 15: 1–2.

Gustafsson, Per: *A World Galloping into Breathlessness. Respiration.* 2001; 69: 2–3.

Hoidal, J. R.: *Genetics of COPD: Present and Future. Europ Resp J.* 2001; 18: 741–43.

Living with COPD. American Lung Association Pamphlet, 1997.

Lockey, Richard F.: *The Basic Principles of Asthma Management Today. J Resp Dis.* (Supp.) 1998; 19: 8–13.

Luskin, M.: *Environmental Control: Key to Asthma Management. J Resp Dis.* 1995; 16: 253–66.

Machin, Odalys, et al: *Confronting the Challenge of Aspirin Induced Asthma. J Resp Dis.* 2001; 22: 625–34.

O'Connell, Edward J., et al: *Cough-Type Asthma. Ann of Allergy.* 1991; 66: 278–82.

Peters, Jay, et al: *Asthma Exacerbations: Key Points from the NIH Guidelines. J Resp Dis.* 1998; 19 (No. 4, April).

Petty, Thomas, ed.: *Chronic Obstructive Pulmonary Disease.* Marcel Dekker, Inc. (New York), 1978.

Prezant, David, et al: *Cough and Bronchial Responsiveness in Firefighters at the World Trade Center Site. N Engl J Med.* 2002; 347: 806–15.

Rits, Thomas, et al: *Emotions and Stress Increase Respiratory Resistance in Asthma. Psychosomatic Medicine.* 2000; 62: 401–12.

Romanik, Katherine: *Around the Clock with COPD.* American Lung Association Pamphlet.

Schachter, Neil: *The Diagnosis and Treatment of Asthma.* Cyberounds. www.Cyberounds.com

Schachter, Neil. *Management of Asthma. The Letter and the Spirit of the New Guidelines.* Cyberounds. www.Cyberounds.com

Sockrider, Marianna, et al: *Environmental Tobacco Smoke: A Real and Present Danger. J Resp Dis.* 15 (No. 8, Aug.), 1994.

Soriano, J.: *Recent Trends in Physician Diagnosed COPD in Women and Men in the UK. Thorax.* 2000; 55: 789–94.

Stevenson, Donald: *Sulfites and Asthma. J Allergy Clin Immunol.* 1984; 72: 469–72.

Storms, W. William: *Exercise Induced Asthma: Making the Diagnosis. J Resp Dis.* 21 (No. 8, Aug.), 2000.

The Asthma Handbook. ALA Pamphlet, 5/98.

The Worldwide Asthma Epidemic: What Can Be Done? Internal Medicine World Report. 16 (No. 11, Sept., Supp.), 2001.

Turato, Graziella, et al: *Pathogenesis and Pathology of COPD. Respiration.* 2001; 68: 117–18.

Viegi, G: *Epidemiology of Chronic Obstructive Pulmonary Disease. Respiration* 2001; 68: 4–19.

Weiland, Jeffrey: *The Differential Diagnosis of COPD and Asthma. Journal of COPD Management.* 2000; Vol. 1; No. 1.

CHAPTER 4

Barnes, P. J.: *New Concepts in the Pathogenesis of Bronchial Hyper-Responsiveness and Asthma. J Allergy Clin Immunol.* 1989; 83: 1013–26.

Didemente, Carlo C., et al: *The Psychology of Smoking Cessation: Helping Smokers Through the Process. Journal of COPD Management.* Vol. 2; No. 4, Oct. 2001.

Donaldson, G. C., et al: *Excess Winter Mortality: Influenza or Cold Stress? Observational Study. BMJ.* 2002; 324: 89–90.

Facts About Home Control of Allergies and Asthma: ALA Pamphlet, 12/97.

Gilliland, F. D., et al: *Effects of Maternal Smoking During Pregnancy and Environmental Tobacco Smoke on Asthma and Wheezing in Children. Am J Respir Crit Care Med.* 2001; 163: 429–36.

Global Strategy for Diagnosis, Management and Prevention of COPD. NHBLI/WHO Workshop Report. Executive Summary. March 2001.

Heinonen, Olli P., et al: *The Effect of Vitamin E and Beta Carotene on the Incidence of Lung Cancer and Other Cancers in Male Smokers. N Engl J Med.* 1994; 330: 1029–34.

Hensley, Michael, et al: *Clinical Epidemiology of COPD.* Marcel Dekker, Inc., (New York), 1989.

Holland, W. W., et al: *Health Effects of Particulate Pollution: Reappraising the Evidence. Am J Epidemiology.* 1979; 110: 527–659.

Kelly, Frank, et al: *Altered Lung Anti-Oxidant Status in Patients with Mild Asthma. The Lancet.* 1999; 354: 482–83.

Koyama, Hiroshi, et al: *Genes, Oxidative Stress and the Risk of Chronic Obstructive Pulmonary Disease. Thorax.* 1998; 53 (Supp.): 510–14.

Mohesenhin, V., et al: *Effects of Ascorbic Acid on the Response to Methacholine Challenge in Asthmatic Subjects. Amer Rev Respir Dis.* 1983; 127: 143–47.

Pauwels, R.: *Global Initiative for Chronic Obstructive Lung Diseases (GOLD): Time to Act. Eur Respir J.* 2001; 18: 901–2.

Piquette, Craig A.: *Exacerbations of COPD: Evaluation and Treatment. J Respir Dis.* Vol. 21; No. 12 (Dec.), 2000.

Powell, Colin, et al: *Antioxidant Status in Asthma. Pediatric Pulmonology.* 1994; 18: 34–38.

Pratico, Domeico, et al: *COPD Associated with an Increase in Urinary Levels of Isoprostone, an Index of Oxidant Stress. Amer J Respir Crit Care Med.* 1998; 158: 1709–14.

Rahmon, Irfon: *Is There Any Relationship Between Plasma Anti-Oxidant Capacity and Lung Function in Smokers and Patients with COPD? Thorax.* 2000; 55: 189–93.

Ries, Andrew: *Preventing COPD: You Can Make a Difference. J Resp Dis.* 1993; 14: 739–49.

Roche, N: *Guidelines versus Clinical Practice in the Treatment of COPD. Eur Respir J.* 2001; 18: 903–8.

Rutgers, SR, et al: *Ongoing Airway Inflammation in Patients with COPD Who Do Not Currently Smoke. Thorax.* 2000; 55: 12–18.

Samet, J. M., et al: *Effect of Anti-Oxidant Supplementation on Ozone-Induced Lung Injury. Am J Respir Crit Care Med.* 2001; 164: 819–25.

Sandberg, S., et al: *The Role of Acute and Chronic Stress in Asthma Attacks in Children. The Lancet.* 2000; 356: 982–87.

Schachter, E. N., et al: *The Attenuation of Exercise-Induced Bronchospasm by Ascorbic Acid. Ann Allergy.* 1982; 49: 146–51.

Schachter, Neil: *Occupational Airway Disease.* Cyberounds.
www.Cyberounds.com

Schachter, Neil: *Programmed Emphysema.* Cyberounds.
www.Cyberounds.com

Shapiro, Steven, et al: *End Stage COPD. Am J Respir Crit Care Med.* 2001; 164: 339–40.

CHAPTER 5

Gibbons, J., et al: *The Significance of Pulmonary Function Testing. Journal of COPD Management.* Vol. 2; No. 5, 2001.

Maguire, George P., et al: *How-and-Why to Use Spirometry in Your Office. J Resp Dis.* Vol. 15; No. 9, Sept., 1994.

National COPD Awareness Panel: *Keys to the Early Detection and Management of COPD. J Resp Dis.* Vol. 21; No. 8, Aug., 2000.

Ryu, Jay, et al: *Obstructive Lung Diseases: Asthma and Many Imitators. Mayo Clin Proc.* 2001; 76: 1144–53.

Standards for the Diagnosis and Care of Patients with COPD. Amer J Respir Crit Care Med. 1995; 152: No. 5 (Nov.).

CHAPTER 6

Baker, J. C., et al: *Diet and Asthma. Respir Med.* 2000; 94: 925–34.

Belloni, Paula, et al: *Effects of All-Trans-Retinoic Acid in Promoting Alveolar Repair, Chest.* 2000; 117: 235S–241S.

Bretton, John, et al: *Dietary Magnesium, Lung Function, Wheezing and Airway Hyperactivity in a Random Adult Population Sample. The Lancet.* 1994; 344: 357–62.

Britton, John: *Dietary Antioxidant Vitamin Intake and a Lung Function in the General Population. Am J Respir Crit Care Med.* 1995; 151: 1383–87.

Britton, John, et al: *Dietary Sodium Intake and the Risk of Airway Hyperactivity in a Random Adult Population. Thorax.* 1994; 49: 875–80.

Burney, P.: *A Diet Rich in Sodium May Potentiate Asthma: Epidemiological Evidence for a New Hypothesis. Chest.* 1987; 91: 143S–148S.

Carey, Oliver, et al: *Effect of Alterations of Dietary Sodium on the Severity of Asthma in Men, Thorax.* 1993; 48: 714–18.

Devereux, Graham, et al: *Effect of Dietary Sodium on Airways Responsiveness and Its Importance in the Epidemiology of Asthma: An Evaluation in Three Areas in Northern England. Thorax.* 1995; 50: 941–47.

Dinsmoor, Robert: *Obesity and Asthma: Is There a Connection? Asthma Magazine.* 27–28, Jan. 2002.

Fogarty, J., et al: *The Role of Diet in the Aetiology of Asthma. Clin Exp Allergy.* 2000; 30: 615–17.

Greene, Lawrence: *Asthma, Oxidant Stress and Diet. Nutrition.* 1999; 15: 899–907.

Hajjar, Ihab, et al: *Impact of Diet on Blood Pressure and Age Related Changes in Blood Pressure in the US Population. Arch Intern Med.* 2001; 161: 589–93.

Hu, Guzhan, et al: *Antioxidant Nutrients and Pulmonary Function: The Third National Health and Nutrition Examination Survey (NHANES III). Am J Epidemiology.* 2000; 151: 975–1316.

Hu, G., et al: *Dietary Vitamin C Intake and Lung Function in Rural China. Am J Epidemiology.* 1998; 148: 594–99.

Knox, Alan. *Salt and Asthma. BMJ.* 1993; 307: 1159–60.

Massaro, G. D., et al: *Retinoic Acid Treatment Abrogates Elastase-Induced Pulmonary Emphysema in Rats. Nature Med.* 1997; 3: 675–77.

Medici, Tullio, et al: *Are Asthmatics Salt Sensitive? Chest.* 1993; 104: 1138–43.

Messerli, Franz: *Salt and Hypertension. Arch Intern Med.* 2001; 161: 505–6.

Miedema, I.: *Dietary Determinants of Long-Term Incidence of Chronic Non-specific Lung Diseases: The Zutphen Study. Am J Epidemiology.* 1993; 138: 37–45.

Mohsenin, Vahid. *Vitamin C and Airways. Annals of New York Academy of Sciences.* 1987; 498: 259–68.

Moore, T. J., et al: *The Dietary Approaches to Stop Hypertension Diet Lowered Systolic Blood Pressure in Stage 1 Isolated Hypertension. Hypertension.* 2001; 38: 155–58.

Morabis, A., et al: *Serum Retinol and Airway Obstruction. Am J Epidemiology.* 1990; 132: 77–82.

Neuman, I., et al: *Reduction of Exercise-Induced Oxidative Stress by Lycopene, a Natural Anti-oxidant. Allergy.* 2000; 55: 1184–89.

Paiva, Sergio, et al: *Assessment of Vitamin A Status in Chronic Obstructive Pulmonary Disease Patients and Healthy Smokers. Am J Clin Nutr.* 1996; 64: 928–34.

Parm, Jonathan: *Effect of Dietary Supplementation with Fish Oil Lipids on Mild Asthma. Thorax.* 1988; 43: 84–92.

Picardo, C., et al: *Dietary Micronutrients/Antioxidants and Their Relationship with Bronchial Asthma Severity. Allergy.* 2001; 56: 43–49.

Pruthi, Sandhya, et al: *Vitamin E Supplementation in the Prevention of Coronary Heart Disease. Mayo Clin Proc.* 2001; 76: 1131–36.

Rahman, Irfan: *Is There Any Relationship Between Plasma Antioxidant Capacity and Lung Function in Smokers and in Patients with COPD? Thorax.* 2000; 55: 189–93.

Rautalahti, Matti, et al: *The Effects of Alpha-Tocopherol and Beta Carotene Supplementation on COPD Symptoms. Am J Respir Crit Care Med.* 1997; 156: 1447–52.

Sacks, Frank, et al: *Effects on Blood Pressure of Reduced Dietary Sodium and the Dietary Approaches to Stop Hypertension (DASH) Diet. N Engl J Med.* 2001; 344: 3–10.

Sargeant, L. A.: *Interaction of Vitamin C with the Relations Between Smoking and Obstructive Disease in Epic, Norfolk. Eur Respir J.* 2000; 16: 397–403.

Schwartz, Joel, et al: *Dietary Factors and their Relation to Respiratory Symptoms. Am J Epidemiology.* 1990; 132: 132–76.

Shahar, Eyal, et al: *Dietary N 3 Polyunsaturated Fatty Acids and Smoking-Related Disease. N Engl J Med.* 1994; 331: 228–33.

Smit, Henriette: *Chronic Obstructive Pulmonary Disease, Asthma and Protective Effects of Food Intake: From Hypothesis to Evidence? Respir Res.* 2001; 2: 261–64.

Smit, Henriette: *Dietary Influences on COPD and Asthma: A Review of the Epidemiological Evidence. Proc Nutr Soc.* 1999; 58: 309–19.

Sridhar, Mongalam: *Clinical Nutrition and Metabolism Group Symposium on "Nutrition and Lung Health." Proc Nutr Soc.* 1999; 58: 303–8.

Stephenson, John: *Experts Air New Findings on Lung Diseases. JAMA.* 1998; 279: 1681–83.

Tabak, Cora, et al: *Dietary Factors and Pulmonary Function: A Cross-Sectional Study in Middle-Aged Men from Three European Countries. Thorax.* 1999; 54: 1021–26.

Tabak, C., et al: *Diet and Chronic Effect of Pulmonary Disease: Independent Beneficial Effects of Fruits, Whole Grains and Alcohol (The Morgan Study). Clin Exp Allergy.* 2001; 31: 747–55.

Trenga, Carol, et al: *Dietary Antioxidants and Ozone Induced Bronchial Hyperresponsiveness in Adults with Asthma. Archives of Environmental Health.* 2001; 56: 242–49.

Tribe, Rachel M., et al: *Dietary Sodium Intake Airway Responsiveness and Cellular Sodium Transport. Am J Respir Crit Care Med.* 1994; 149: 1426–33.

Virtamo, Jarmo: *Vitamins and Cancer. Proc Nutr Soc.* 1999; 58: 329–33.

Vollmer, William, et al: *Effects of Diet and Sodium Intake on Blood Pressure: Subgroup Analysis of the DASH Sodium Trial. Ann Intern Med.* 2001; 135: 1020–28.

Wang, Zengquan, et al: *Ultraviolet Irradiation of Human Skin Causes Functional Vitamin A Deficiency Preventable by All Transretinoic Acid Pretreatment. Nature Medicine.* 1999; 5: 418–22.

Willett, Walter: *What Vitamins Should I Be Taking, Doctor? N Engl J Med.* 2001; 345: 1819–24.

Yemaneberhan, Haile, et al: *Prevalence of Wheeze and Asthma and Relation to Atrophy in Urban and Rural Ethiopia. The Lancet.* 1997; 350: 85–90.

CHAPTER 7

ACCP/AACVPR Pulmonary Rehabilitation Guidelines Panel: *Pulmonary Rehabilitation. Chest.* 1997; 112: 1363–96.

Alliverti, Andrea: *How and Why Exercise Is Impaired in COPD. Respiration.* 2001; 63: 229–39.

ATS Board of Directors: *Pulmonary Rehabilitation 1999. Am J Respir Crit Care Med.* 1999; 159: 1666–82.

Bach, John (ed.): *Pulmonary Rehabilitation.* Hanley and Belfurs (Philadelphia), 1996.

Bannister, Roger: *Sport, Physical Reaction and the National Health. Brit Med Jour.* 1972; 4: 711–15.

Beck, Kenneth: *Control of Airway Function During and After Exercise in Asthmatics. Medical Science in Sports and Exercise,* 1999.

Cambach, W., et al: *The Effects of a Community Based Pulmonary Rehabilitation Programe on Exercise Tolerance and Quality of Life: A Randomized Controlled Trial. Eur Respir J.* 1997; 10: 104–13.

Clark, Christopher, et al: *Assessment of Work Performance in Asthma for Determination of Cardiorespiratory Fitness and Training Capacity. Thorax.* 1988; 43: 745–49.

D'Alessandro, Allessandra: *Exaggerated Response to Choline Inhalation Among Persons with Non-specific Airway Hyperactivity. Chest.* 1996; 109: 331–37.

Fowler, Christopher: *Preventing and Managing Exercise-Induced Asthma. Asthma Magazine.* pp. 25–35, March 2001.

Garfinkel, S. K.: *Physiologic and Nonphysiologic Determinants of Aerobic Fitness in Mild to Moderate Asthma. Am Rev Respir Dis.* 1992; 145: 741–45.

Haas, Francois, et al: *Effect of Aerobic Training Forced Expiratory Airflow in Exercising Asthmatic Humans. J Appl Physiol.* 1987; 63: 1230–35.

Henriksen, J. M., et al: *Effect of Physical Training on Exercise-Induced Bronchoconstriction. Acta Paediatr Scand.* 1983; 72: 31–36.

Hensen, Ejvind, et al: *Reversible and Irreversible Air Flow Obstruction as Predictor of Overall Mortality in Asthma and COPD. Am J Respir Crit Care Med.* 1999; 159: 1267–71.

Hsia, Connie: *Cardiopulmonary Limitations to Exercise in Restrictive Lung Disease. Medicine and Science in Sports and Exercise,* 1999.

Kurabayashi, Hitoshi, et al: *Effective Physical Therapy for COPD. Am J Phys Med Rehabil.* 1997; 76: 204–7.

Lakka, T. A.: *Exercise and Heart Disease: More Good Reasons to Get in Shape. N Engl J Med.* 1994; 330: 1549–54.

Larson, Janet: *Cycle Ergometer and Inspiratory Muscle Training in COPD. Am J Respir Crit Care Med.* 1999; 100: 500–7.

Leermakers, Elizabeth: *Exercise Management of Obesity. Medical Clinics of North America.* 2000; 84: 419–39.

Leith, David: *Ventilatory Muscle Strength and Endurance Training. J Appl Phys.* 1976; 41: 508–15.

McFadden, E. R., Jr.: *Exercise-Induced Airway Obstruction. Clinics in Chest Medicine.* 1995; 16: 671–82.

Niederman, Michael, et al: *Benefits of Multidisciplinary Pulmonary Rehabilitation Program. Chest.* 1992; 99: 798–904.

O'Donnell, Denis E.: *Spirometric Correlates of Improvement in Exercise Performance after Anticholinergic Therapy in COPD. Am J Respir Crit Care Med.* 1999; 160: 542–49.

Randolph, Christopher: *Exercise-Induced Asthma: Update on Pathophysiology, Clinical Diagnosis and Treatment. Current Problems in Pediatrics.* Feb., 53–77, 1997.

Ringsbaek, T. J., et al: *Rehabilitation of Patients with Chronic Obstructive Pul-*

monary Disease—Exercise Twice a Week Is Not Sufficient! Respiratory Medicine. 2000; 94: 150–54.

Roger, Nuria: *Nitric Oxide Inhalation During Exercise in COPD. Am J Respir Crit Care Med.* 1997; 156: 800–6.

Storms, William: *Exercise-Induced Asthma: Diagnosis and Treatment for the Recreational or Elite Athlete. Medicine and Science in Sports and Exercise.* 1999.

Sue, Darryl, et al: *Impact of Integrative Cardiopulmonary Exercise Testing on Clinical Decision Making. Chest.* 1991; 99: 981–82.

Yan, Sheng, et al: *Inspiratory Muscle Mechanics of Patients with COPD During Incremental Exercise. Am J Respir Crit Care Med.* 1997; 156: 807–13.

ZuWallack, Richard, et al: *Predictors of Improvements in the 1 Minute Walking Distance Following a Six Week Out Patient Pulmonary Rehabilitation Program. Chest.* 1991; 99: 805–8.

CHAPTER 8

ATS Board of Directors Official Statement on Cigarette Smoking and Health. Am J Respir Crit Care Med. 1996; 153: 861–65.

Boschert, Sherry: *Sustained-Release Bupropion Aids Smoking Cessation in COPD. Internal Medicine News.* Feb. 15, page 33, 2001.

Bretton, John: *Helping People to Stop Smoking: The New Smoking Cessation Guidelines. Thorax.* 1999; 54: 1–2.

Brown, Phyllida: *Tobacco Smoke Kills One Smoker in Two. New Scientist.* 1994; 15: 4.

Dale, Lowell, et al: *Treatment of Nicotine Dependence. Mayo Clin Proc.* 2000; 75: 1311–16.

Fontham, E. T. H., et al: *Passive Smoke: Clear Risk Factor for Lung Cancer No Matter What the Source. JAMA.* 1994; 271: 1752–59.

Goldman, Erik: *After Acute MI, 22% of Female Smokers Got the Nicotine Patch. Internal Medicine News.* Dec. 15, 2001.

Harmanjatinder, S. S., et al: *Prenatal Nicotine Exposure Alters Pulmonary Function in Newborn Rhesus Monkeys. Am J Respir Crit Care Med.* 2001; 164: 989–94.

Hays, J. Taylor, et al: *Sustained Release Bupropion for Pharmacologic Relapse Prevention After Smoking Cessation. Ann Intern Med.* 2001; 135: 423–33.

Howell, Donna: *The Unofficial Guide to Quitting Smoking.* IDG Books World-wide, 2000.

Iribarren, Carlos, et al: *Effect of Cigar Smoking on the Risk of Cardiovascular Disease, COPD, and Cancer in Men. N Engl J Med.* 2001; 340: 1773–80.

Mazurek, Douglas, et al: *Smoking Cessation Lessons from the Lung Health Study. J Resp Dis.* 1995; 16: 1049–60.

Wilson, Clare: *My Friend Nicotine. New Scientist.* Nov. 10, pp. 28–31, 2001.

CHAPTER 9

Adams, Sandra: *Treating Acute Exacerbations of Chronic Bronchitis in the Face of Antibiotic Resistance. Clev Clin J Med.* 2000; 67: 625–32.

Appelbaum, Peter, et al: *Declining Antibiotic Susceptibility Among Respiratory Tract Pathogens. J Resp Dis.* 2001; 22: 19–25.

Beakes, Douglas: *The Use of Anticholinergics in Asthma. Journal of Asthma.* 1997; 34: 357–68.

Benowitz, N. L., et al: *What to Tell Patients with Heart Disease About Nicotine Therapy. J Amer Coll Cardiol.* 1997; 29: 1422–31.

Brostoff, Johnathan, et al: *The Complete Guide to Integrative Therapies.* Healing Arts Press (Rochester), 2000.

Cave, A.: *Inhaled and Nasal Corticosteroids: Factors Affecting the Risks of Systemic Adverse Effects. Pharmacol Ther.* Sept. 1999; 83(3): 153–79.

Dennis, S. M., et al: *Regular Inhaled Salbutamol: The TRUST Randomized Trial. The Lancet.* 2000; 355: 1675–79.

Global Initiative for Asthma. *Global Strategy for Asthma Management and Prevention.* Bethesda, MD; NIH.1995, NHLBI/WHO Workshop Report. Publication #95–3659.

Gross, Nicholas: *How to Manage Acute Exacerbations of COPD. J Resp Dis.* 2001; 22: 65–68.

Gross, Nicholas, et al: *Optimal Treatment for COPD. Patient Care.* May 30, 2000.

Huntley, A., et al: *Relaxation Therapies for Asthma. Thorax.* 2002; 57: 127–31.

Jick, S. S., et al: *The Risk of Cataracts Among Users of Inhaled Steroids. Epidemiology.* March 2001; 12 (2): 228–34.

Lazarus, S. C., et al: *Long-Acting Beta Agonist Monotherapy vs. Continued Ther-

apy with Inhaled Corticosteroids in Patients with Persistent Asthma. JAMA. 2001; 285: 2583–93.

Lung Health Study Research Group: *Effects of Inhaled Triamcinolone on the Decline of Pulmonary Function in COPD. N Engl J Med.* 2000; 343: 1902–9.

McEvoy, Charlene, et al: *Association Between Corticosteroid Use and Vertebral Fractures in Older Men with COPD. Am J Respir Crit Care Med.* 1998; 157: 704–9.

Moser, M. R.: *An Outbreak of Influenza Aboard a Commercial Airliner. Amer J Epidemiology.* 1979; 110: 1–6.

National Asthma Education and Prevention Program. Expert Panel Report 2: *Guidelines for the Diagnosis and Management of Asthma.* Bethesda, MD: National Institutes of Health; 1997. NIH publication #97–4051.

Nelson, H. S.: *Clinical Experience with Levalbuterol. J Allergy Clin Immunol.* 1999; 104 (2 pt. 2): 577–84.

Olson, C. G., et al: *Is Your Patient's Cough Due to an ACE Inhibitor. Arch Fam Med.* 1995; 4: 525–28.

Pol, Robert: *Theophylline: Still a Reasonable Choice. J Resp Dis.* 1994; 15: 19–32.

Poole, P. J.: *Oral Mucolytic Drugs for Exacerbation of COPD. BMJ;* 2001; 322: 1271–74.

Radimir, Kathy L.: *Non Vitamin, Non Mineral Dietary Supplements: Issues and Findings. J of the Amer Diet Assoc.* 2000; 100: 447–54.

San Pedro, Gerardo: *Treating Acute Exacerbations of Acute Bronchitis. Hospital Practice.* Nov. 15, 2000; 43–50.

Sklon, David, et al: *Inhibition of the Activity of Human Leukocyte Elastase by Lipid Oleic Acid and Retinoic Acid. Lung.* 1990; 168: 323–32.

Toogood, J. H.: *Side Effects of Inhaled Corticosteroids. J Allergy Clin Immunol.* 1998; 102: 705–13.

Tsukagoshi, H., et al: *Evidence of Oxidative Stress on Asthma and COPD: Potential Inhibitory Effect of Theophylline. Respir Med.* 2000; 94: 584–88.

Walsh, L. J., et al: *Adverse Effects of Oral Corticosteroids in Relation to Dose in Patients with Lung Disease. Thorax.* 2001, Apr; 56 (4): 279–84.

Witek, T. J., Schachter, E. N.: *Pharmacology and Therapeutics in Respiratory Care.* Saunders (Philadelphia). 1994.

Wong, C. A., et al: *Inhaled Corticosteroid Use and Bone-Mineral Density in Patients with Asthma. The Lancet.* 2000. 355: 1399–1403.

Woolcock, A.: *Effects of Inhaled Corticosteroids on Bone Density and Metabolism. J Allergy Clin Immunol.* 1998; 101: S456–59.

Ziment, Irwin: *How Your Patients May Be Using Herbalism to Treat Their Asthma. J Resp Dis.* 1998; 19: 1070–81.

Ziment, Irwin: *What Else Are Your Patients Using to Treat their Asthma. J Resp Dis.* 1999; 20: 58–64.

CHAPTER 10

Bruce, N., et al: *Indoor Air Pollution in Developing Countries: A Major Environmental and Public Health Challenge. Bull World Health Organization.* 2000; 78: 1078–92.

Chan-Yeung, Moira: *Effectiveness and Compliance to Intervention Measures in Reducing House Dust and Cat Allergen Levels. Ann Allergy, Asthma Immunol.* 2002; 88: 52–58.

Crawford, John: *How Serious Is Sick Building Syndrome? Advance.* March 2002, p. 34–37.

Custovic A., et al: *Clinical Effects of Allergen Avoidance. Clin Review Allerg Immunol.* 2000; 18: 397–419.

Dorward, A. J.: *Effect of House Mite Avoidance Measures on Adult Atopic Asthma. Thorax.* 1988; 43: 98–102.

Godfrey, K.: *House Dust Mite Avoidance—The Way Forward. Clin Exp Allergy.* 1991; 21: 1–2.

Johanning, E., et al: *Building Related Illnesses Associated with Moisture and Fungal Contamination: Current Concepts. N Engl J Med.* 1998; 338: 1070.

Jones, A. P.: *Asthma and the Home Environment. J Asthma.* April 2000 (Review).

Knust, F. M.: *House Dust Mite Avoidance—The Right Way to Go Forward. Clin Exp Allergy.* 1992; 22: 589–90.

Kreiss, K.: *The Sick Building Syndrome: Where Is the Epidemiological Basis? Amer J Pub Health.* 1990; 80: 1172–73.

Marks, S. B.: *House Dust Mite Exposure as a Risk Factor for Asthma: Benefits of Avoidance. Allergy.* 1998; 53: 108–14.

Menzies, D., et al: *Building Related Illness. N Engl J Med.* 1997; 337: 1524–31.

Murray, A. B.: *Dust-Free Bedrooms in the Treatment of Asthmatic Children with House Dust or House Dust Mite Allergy: A Controlled Trial. Pediatrics.* 1983; 71: 418–22.

Peat, J. K.: *Effects of Damp and Mold in the Homes on Respiratory Health: A Review. Allergy.* 1998; 53: 120–28.

Redlich, C. A., et al: *Sick Building Syndrome. The Lancet.* 1997; 349: 1013–16.

Sheikh, A., et al: *House Mite Avoidance Measures for Perennial Allergic Rhinitis. Cochrane Database Syst. Rev.* Vol. 4; 2001.

Smet, J. M., et al: *Health Effects and Sources of Indoor Air Pollution. Pt. 2. Amer Rev Respir Dis.* 1988; 1137: 221–42.

Witek, T. J., Schachter, E. N. (eds.): *Problems in Respiratory Care Parts I and II.* Lippincott (Philadelphia), 1990.

CHAPTER 11

Bartsch, Peter: *High Altitude Pulmonary Edema. Medicine and Science in Sports and Exercise.* 1999; 31: S23–S27.

Bascom, Rebecca: *Health Effects of Outdoor Air Pollution. Am J Respir Crit Care Med.* 1996; 153: 3–50.

Benjamin, Berg, et al: *Oxygen Supplementation During Air Travel in Patients with COPD. Chest.* 1992; 101: 638–41.

Chan-Yeung, M.: *Occupational Asthma—State of the Art. Am Rev Respir Dis.* 1986; 133: 688–703.

Chapman, Sheila: *Take Wing with Oxygen. Advance.* March 2002, pp. 55–56.

Coker, R. K., et al: *Assessing the Risk of Hypoxia in Flight: The Need for More Rational Guidelines. Eur Respir J.* 2000; 15: 128–30.

Cramer, D., et al: *Assessment of Oxygen Supplementation During Air Travel. Thorax.* 1996; 51: 202–3.

Dillard, Thomas, et al: *Hypoxemia During Air Travel with Patients with COPD. Ann Intern Med.* 1989; 11: 362–67.

Ford, Genie. *The Air Up There. Allergy and Asthma.* Summer 2001, pp. 57–63.

Gong, Henry, et al: *Preflight Medical Screenings of Patients. Chest.* 1993; 104: 788–94.

Horton, D. J., et al: *Effects of Breathing Warm Humidified Air on Bronchoconstric-*

tion Induced by Body Cooling and by Inhalation of Methacholine. *Chest.* 1979;
75: 24.

Horvath, E. P., et al: *Building Related Illness and Sick Building Syndrome—from the Specific to the Vague. Clev Clin J Med.* 1997; 64: 303–9.

Karjalaien, A., et al: *Work Related to Substantial Portion of Adult Onset Asthma Incidence in the Finnish Population. Am J Respir Crit Care Med.* 2001; 164: 565–68.

Laposstolle, Frederic, et al: *Severe Pulmonary Embolism Associated with Air Travel. N Engl J Med.* 2001; 345: 779–83.

Leight, J. P., et al: *Costs of Occupational COPD and Asthma. Chest.* 2002; 21: 264–72.

Lyznicki, James, et al: *Medical Oxygen and Air Travel. Aviation, Space and Environmental Med.* 2000; 71: 827–31.

Stoller, J. K.: *Travel for the Technology Dependent Individual. Respir Care.* 1994; 39: 347–62.

Thiel, H., et al: *Baker's Asthma: Development and Possibility for Treatment. Chest.* 1980 (2 Supp.); 78: 400–5.

Acknowledgments

I would like to acknowledge the support and friendship of:

My colleagues at Mount Sinai: Drs. Alvin Tierstein, Gwen Skloot, David Nierman, Maria Padilla, Phillip Landrigan, Irving Selikoff, Eugenia Zuskin, Judy Nelson, Tom Kalb, Louis Depalo, Cynthia Caracta, Carol Rosenbaum, and Chris Cardozo.

The staff and board members of the American Lung Association of the City of New York: Cynthia Erickson, our extraordinary CEO, Louise Leavitt, my friend and mentor Robert Mellins, MD, Bernadette Murphy, Bill Daughtry, Jack Pasini, Rob Roth, James Smith, MD, David Rapoport, MD, Joan Reibman, MD, and Randi Fain, MD.

The incredible staff at Mount Sinai: My friend and right arm, Theo Hoke, Lourdes Mateo, Judy Schneiderman, Shirley Palleja, Denise Williams, Deya Jourdy, Uma Arumagam and Nick Rienzi.

The doctors who generously gave their time and assistance: Neil Schluger, MD, of Columbia Presbyterian Hospital,

Johnathan Raskin, MD, of Beth Israel North Hospital, Noah Greenspan of the Pulmonary Wellness and Rehabilitation Center, and Meyer Kattan, MD, Chief of Pediatric Pulmonary Medicine at Mount Sinai Medical Center.

My colleagues from Yale University: Herbert Reynolds, MD, now Chief of Medicine at Hershey Medical Center, Arend Bouyhus, MD, Ph.D, the late Chief of Pulmonary Medicine, Arthur Dubois, MD, of the Pierce Foundation at Yale, Michael Littner, MD, Theodore Witek, Ph.D, now with Boehringer Ingelheim, Michael Niederman, MD, now Chief of Pulmonary Medicine at Winthrop University Hospital and Richard Matthay, MD, Vice Chairman of Medicine at Yale University School of Medicine, and Samuel O. Thier, MD, former Chief of Medicine at Yale.

My teachers and colleagues at NYU Medical Center: The late John McClement, MD, Saul Farber, MD, Martin Kahn, MD, S. Arthur Localio, MD, and Joseph Ransahoff, MD.

To Maria Perez, Joe Montenez, and Mark Glackin from GlaxoSmithKline, whose support has helped the American Lung Association of the City of New York to reach out and raise awareness of asthma and COPD.

To my agent extraordinaire Marly Rousoff, whose intelligence and support shaped my general ideas into a real book, and then has stayed with me to smooth the journey to publication.

My very smart and patient editor Gerald Howard, publisher of Broadway Books, whose insight, skill, and commitment developed a book that provides lifesaving advice in a tone and style that people can actually understand.

My fellow soldiers in the battle with the tobacco industry

and environmental health: Joe Cherner, founder of SmokeFree Educational Services, Hubert Humphrey III, former governor of Minnesota, Ira Burnim of the Southern Povery Law Office, and Eric Frumin of A.C.T.W.U.

My artists Elizabeth Sample and Eric Faltreco, for the beautiful work they did on the medical illustrations.

My fellow pulmonologists: Peter Barnes of the National Heart and Lung Institute in London, Nicholas Gross, MD, of the Stitch School of Medicine of Loyola University, Dean Hess, RRT, of Massachusetts General Hospital, and Neil MacIntyre, MD, of Duke University.

Finally, I want to thank my wife Deborah Chase for her tolerance, as well as her very considerable editorial and promotional support, my daughters, Karen and Lauren for their love and patience, and Martha and Allen Chase for allowing me to join their family.

Index

Index

tidal volume, 25
See also shortness of breath
bronchitis
  COPD and, 6
  coughing up blood with, 78–79
  mucus plugs and, 26
  neutrophils and, 27–28
  rhonchi, 87
  vitamin C and, 106
  See also chronic bronchitis
bronchodilators, 93–94, 177–82, 188
  anticholinergic, 180–82
  beta agonists, 177–78
  beta agonists, long-acting, 179–80
  beta agonists, short-acting, 177,
    178–79
bronchoscopy, 211

CAT scan, 36, 98–99
Ceclor, 191
Ceftin, 191
chest pain, 77–78
chest workup
  blood tests, 99–101
  bronchodilator test, 93–94
  cardiac examination, 89
  CAT scan, 98–99
  chest X ray, 90
  diffusion capacity test, 95
  exercise, 101–2
  family history, 84–85
  methacholine test, 94–95
  nuclear scans, 102–3
  past medical history, 79–84
  physical exam, 85–90
  plethysmograph, *97*, 98
  pulse oximetry test, 96–97, *96*
  smoking history, 80–83
  spirometry for testing lung
    function, 91–93, *91*, 95
  symptoms, 75–79
  testing, 90–103
cholesterol, 109–10, 132
chronic bronchitis, 30–32, *31*
  diagnosis, 31
  emphysema with, 36

smoking and, 32
treatment, 182
workplace pollution and, 32
Cipro, 192
climate, 12, 271–72
colds and flu
  antibiotics and, 49, 190–93
  antiviral medication, 189–90
  flu shots, 189, 190, 281
COPD (chronic obstructive
    pulmonary disease)
  alternative strategies, 12
  antioxidants and, 9
  asthma and, 5–6, 49–51
  bronchitis and, 6
  care strategies, 6, 8
  causes, 8, 10, 264–65
  delay in seeking help, consequences
    of, 4, 12–13, 29–30
  denial, 79–80
  diagnosis, 13
  diagnosis, second opinions, 268
  diet and, 6, 9
  emphysema and, 6
  genetics and, 36–37, 264–65, 267
  heart failure and, 38
  heart problems and, 88–90
  irreversible pulmonary constriction
    and, 6
  lung function, conditions affecting,
    26
  lung function decline and, 6
  medical specialty for, 268
  medication for, 8, 11
  preventive strategies, 11
  residual volume increase, 25
  rising incidence of, 2–3, 158,
    266–67
  risk questionnaire, 7
  smoker's cough and, 8
  smoking and, 1–2, 6, 54–57
  Stage 0, 37–38
  Stage I, 38
  Stage II, 38
  Stage III, 38–39
  statistics, 2, 29

Levaquin, 192
lung
  alveoli, *17*, 18, 21, 26, 33–34, *33*,
    58, 95
  asthma, and damage to, 43–44
  biochemical functions, 26–28
  bronchi, *15*, 16–17, 31–32, *31*
  care strategies and understanding
    anatomy and function, 14
  cells, goblet, 20
  cells, pseudostratified columnar
    epithelium, 19, 20, 68
  cells, Type I, 20–21
  cells, Type II, 21
  cilia, 19, 20, 27, 68
  collapsed, 25
  COPD and function decline, 6,
    267–68
  dynamic lung function, 25–26
  elastin, 18, 34, 57, 58–59
  exchange-diffusion function, 26
  function, 4, 267–68
  immunologic function, 27–28
  lobes, 16
  mucus, 19–20
  muscles of respiration, 24
  obesity and oxidative stress, 10
  overexpansion (emphysema),
    18–19
  pleura, 16
  pollutants, fatal four, 68–74
  pulmonary system, design and
    function, 15–28, *15, 17, 22*
  quiet, 87–88
  remodeling, 43, 58, 67
  residual volume (RV), 25
  respiration, process of, 18
  smoker's, 58
  smooth muscle, 19–20, 59, 177
  smooth muscle, constricted, 20
  static lung function, 24–25
  surface area, 17–18
  surfactant, 21
  vital capacity, 25, 209
  X ray, "dirty" appearance, 31
lung cancer, 78, 79, 90

COPD and, 266
  smoking and, 157
lung transplantation, 211–12
lung volume reduction surgery
  (LVRS), 209–11, 266
lycopene, 111

McClement, John, 2–3
Massaro, Gloria and Donald, 109
mediator-modifying drugs, 193–95
  antihistamines, 194
  chromones, 188, 194
  leukotriene blocking agents, 188,
    194
  new, 195
medication. *See* inhalers; treatment;
    specific drugs
meditation, 12, 201–2
methacholine, 94–95

neutrophils, 27–28, 34, 186
NHANES II (Second National Health
    and Nutrition Examination
    Survey), 106
NHANES III (Third National Health
    and Nutrition Examination
    Survey), 109
nosebleeds, 83
Novella, Antonio, 157

obesity, 127–30
  asthma and, 10
oxidative stress
  antioxidants to prevent, 113
  asthma, COPD and, 105, 112
  diet and prevention of, 105
  obesity and, 10
  smoking and, 56, 59
oxygen replacement therapy, 207
  compressed oxygen, 207
  insurance reimbursement, 208
  liquid, 208
  oxygen concentrator, 208

peak flow meter, 50–51, 93
phlegm, 76–77

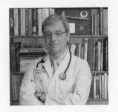

About the Author

Neil Schachter, MD, is Professor of Pulmonary and Community Medicine, Medical Director of the Respiratory Care Department, and Associate Director of the Pulmonary Division of the Mount Sinai Medical Center. Author of five books and more than 400 articles on pulmonary disease, Dr. Schachter is past president of the American Lung Association of the City of New York and the National Association of Medical Directors of Respiratory Care. At Yale University School of Medicine, he was appointed Director of Respiratory Therapy at Yale New Haven Hospital, where he published his landmark research on the role of vitamin C for asthma.